AUTHOR BIO

Suki Bains drew on her own life experiences, analysis and years of education to build the one-of-a-kind programme introduced in *How Do You Feel?* She has taken Holistic training courses and has independently researched subjects like mental health and psychology. Suki has lived in several countries, where she learned to immerse herself into different cultures, and this has given her a unique point of view and the ability to view life from many perspectives. Plus, she has always been an empath, so opening up and exploring emotions is nothing new. And now, she sets out to help you on the same path so that you, too, can get to know yourself on the deepest level – and maintain that important relationship for years to come.

HOW DO YOU FEEL?

**A Holistic Guide to help you to work successfully
with your mental, emotional, physical,
spiritual and whole self**

Suki Bains

First published in Great Britain 2021 by Cherish Editions

Cherish Editions is a trading style of Shaw Callaghan Ltd &
Shaw Callaghan 23 USA, INC.
The Foundation Centre
Navigation House, 48 Millgate, Newark
Nottinghamshire NG24 4TS UK
www.triggerhub.org
Text Copyright © 2021 Suki Bains

British Library Cataloguing in Publication Data
A CIP catalogue record for this book is available upon request from the
British Library
ISBN: 978-1-913615-35-2
Suki Bains has asserted her right under the Copyright,
Design and Patents Act 1988 to be identified as the author of this work
Cover design by Moljala Studio, Irene Salo Studio and More Visual
Typeset by Lapiz Digital Services

Cherish Editions encourages diversity and different viewpoints; however, all
views, thoughts, and opinions expressed in this book are the author's own
and are not necessarily representative of Cherish Editions as an organization.

All material in this book is set out in good faith for general guidance
and no liability can be accepted for loss or expense incurred in following
the information given. In particular this book is not intended to replace
expert medical or psychiatric advice. It is intended for informational
purposes only and for your own personal use and guidance. It is not
intended to diagnose, treat or act as a substitute for professional medical
advice. The author is not a medical practitioner nor a counsellor, and
professional advice should be sought if desired before embarking on any
health-related programme.

TABLE OF CONTENTS

Letter from the author   7
Introduction   9

Part 1   **How do you feel?**
                Gaining Awareness   **19**
Chapter 1   How do you feel? All parts of you:
                as a whole   21
Chapter 2   How do you feel? As yourself:
                inside and out   39
Chapter 3   Introduction to the Dictionary of Feelings   55
Chapter 4   Dictionary of Feelings – Positive   63
Chapter 5   Dictionary of Feelings – Neutral   105
Chapter 6   Dictionary of Feelings – Negative   111
Chapter 7   How do you feel as a whole?   187

Part 2   **How to work successfully with**
                your whole self (being practical)   **189**
Chapter 8   How to successfully start working
                with your feelings   191
Chapter 9   How to successfully work
                with your mental self   199
Chapter 10 How to successfully work
                with your emotional self   265

Chapter 11 How to successfully work
with your physical self   297

Chapter 12 How to successfully work
with your spiritual self   323

Chapter 13 How to successfully work
with your whole self   339

LETTER FROM THE AUTHOR

Dear Reader,

You are the only one who will know the truth of what it feels like to be you, inside your mind and body. You are the only one who knows how life feels for you, as you stand where you stand, and experience your life from your perspective, positions and point of view. You are the only one who knows what it is like to have walked your journey of life, in your footsteps, through your stages and phases and changes of your life.

I am very aware no one will know what it is like to be you. It is through your mind, your body, and your spirit that you feel life; it is through your instincts, your senses, and your emotions that you will feel your way through life; and it is through your reactions and actions and through your behaviour that you will bring yourself face to face with life.

However, in life, it is easy to forget who you are, and easy to lose the truth of who you are.

The truth is, there will be days in your life when:

- life will not make sense in your mind
- you will feel bad inside your mind and body
- you will struggle to connect with yourself
- your life will not feel safe or secure or stable
- you will feel stuck – as if you are in a cycle or circle

- you will struggle to align as a whole, inside and out
- you will feel loss, anger, hurt, confusion, conflict and pain
- you will feel emotions and feelings that you cannot name
- you will have to make choices and decisions on your own
- you will walk your journey of life all by yourself
- you will feel isolated and lonely and misunderstood
- you will struggle to process or understand yourself, or even life itself
- the world you are living in will not feel kind or safe; it will feel unsafe
- you will have to go inside yourself and be face to face with yourself

When this happens to you:

- where will you go?
- what will you do?
- who will you turn to?

As you are the only one that can see and feel all parts of you, and you are the only one that can answer the truth of what is happening inside and outside of you, I have written this guide to help you come back to your true self and to help you to work successfully with your whole self:

Mentally: your emotions, thoughts, perceptions and perspective narrative
Emotionally: your emotions and feelings in mind and body
Physically: your reactions, actions and behaviours
Spiritually: your unseen energy, which connects you to life

Suki Bains
May 2021

INTRODUCTION

The goal of this guide

The goal of *How Do You Feel?* is to help you become deeply aware of who you are and how you feel, so you can see your whole self clearly. It is written to help you step inside of yourself first and to see the unseen parts of yourself – your emotions, feelings, thoughts, opinions, judgements and beliefs – which can keep you stuck or struggling, or hold you back in life. If you cannot see and feel these parts, you cannot work successfully with them.

Only when you see your whole self clearly, inside and out, can you start to take steps to work _with_ your whole self rather than _against_ your whole self.

Why have I written this guide?

My desire to create a holistic guide to help you work successfully with your whole self, inside and out, started when I was a child. From an early age, I was aware that I could see and feel another person's hurt, internal struggle and emotional pain that they themselves could not put into words or acknowledge, or that they found hard to reveal. I could see the struggle and pain in their eyes, or through the masked smile, or in the forced posture; I could see it in the words that did not align with the truth of a feeling deep inside. At the same time that I was becoming aware of others, I was also becoming aware of my own emotions and feelings and thoughts, based on all that I was absorbing, seeing and experiencing in life.

I found myself living in a world that was divided and focused on the external alone. It was teaching me who to be, how to be and what to be – but only half of me.

What about the other parts of me?

It was not guiding me on how to work with the unseen part of myself, the part of me that no-one else could see and feel but me.

What about the parts of me that I was left alone at night to deal with?

I wanted to ask:

What is this inside of me?

What is this unseen part of me?

What is this emotion?

What is this thought?

What is this feeling?

What is the part of me you cannot see?

Why are you only teaching me how to work with half of me?

Why not all of me?

TWO WORLDS NEED TO ALIGN

I found myself navigating two worlds. I knew back then that these two worlds – the internal and the external – needed to align. I knew that emotions, feelings, thoughts – no matter how far hidden deep inside of the mind and body – were important in life. I knew it was not healthy to deny or hide them or to push the truth away. I knew we needed to implement a way of learning (a system) to find ways to work successfully with all parts of the self, inside and out. More importantly, I knew that if we did not implement this system or create time and space for this area, it would eventually impact all of us, not only individually, but collectively

THE PAIN AND STRUGGLE

Thirty years later, and so many people around the world are struggling mentally, emotionally, physically and spiritually. Emotions and feelings are being suppressed, rejected, buried, misused, abused, and ignored. People worldwide are either over-expressing, under-expressing, silently suffering or keeping their true feelings inside. There are so many of us who are stuck in fear, anger, anxiety and depression and cannot find a way out. So many struggle to find the words to express how they feel, so they feel alone on this journey of life.

On top of this, we live in an era where the word "feeling" has become uncomfortable to use, and is almost stigmatized. Instead of learning to work successfully with our inner emotions, we turn feelings into words that are wrapped into opinions, judgements, conclusions and beliefs that do not reveal the truth of a feeling underneath. And this is where we often choose to stay – stuck behind these words, which we use to protect or defend or to cut like a sword... and also stuck behind negative reactions, actions and behaviours, which turn the truth of bad feelings from the inside, and manifest in the outside world.

By being this way, not only are we separating ourself from ourself, but we are separating ourselves from one another.

There is a huge gap that lies in between the unseen parts and the seen parts. This is where misunderstanding, conflict and confusion lie and continue to grow over time.

The way we all feel on the inside is manifesting itself on the outside. The world on the outside is divided and polarized, and that is a result of what is happening when we are not aligned, and not working successfully with our whole self – from the inside out.

Something needs to change – there needs to be a new way.

The solution:
An holistic guide, to help you work successfully with yourself, inside and out and as a whole.

THE CALLING

Although I have waited over 30 years to deliver this guide into your hands, the actual calling to write this guide happened over two years ago. There was a voice inside of me that was becoming louder and louder, but I kept avoiding this voice, allowing myself to hide behind fear. Yet, as time passed, and after seeing so much help available via medication, self-help books, and different teachings, I could see that people were still struggling worldwide. I could see the root of the problem had still not been addressed. Then a global pandemic hit, and I felt I had no choice – I had to finally deliver on the promise I made to myself as a child. So I sat down and started to write an holistic guide to heal the root instead of covering up the confusion, conflict and pain.

Why "holistic"?

"Holistic" means to see all parts of yourself as one, with all parts connected, interconnected and linked. And you can apply this to yourself, to others, and to life as a whole. If you see yourself holistically, you are **aware** of yourself as a whole. You will know if one part of you is not working successfully, as it will influence and impact other parts of you to. For example, if you do not look after yourself mentally, this can impact you emotionally; if you do not look after yourself emotionally, it can impact you physically; if you do not look after yourself physically, it can impact you spiritually; and if you do not look after yourself spiritually, it can impact your connection with life and with others.

How this guide will help you

Part 1: How do you feel? Gaining awareness has been written to bring you back to basics – to treat your mind and body as a clean slate. It will help you to step into awareness – to see, know and understand what is happening to you, inside and out.

There are three steps to help you step into awareness:

Step 1: To be aware of all the parts of yourself that make you whole
Step 2: To be aware of your-self and see yourself inside and out
Step 3: To be aware of your emotions and feelings – in mind and body
  Step 3 involves the use of **The Dictionary of Feelings**. The dictionary explains over 140 emotions and feelings.

Each emotion and feeling is broken down as follows:

Name:
Meaning:
Purpose:
Feeling:
What happens inside the body?
What happens outside of the body?
Reaction:
Root:

By providing a name, a meaning, and a purpose for each of your emotions and feelings, the dictionary will help you to:

- move your emotions and feelings from the dark into the light
- see how each emotion and feeling impacts and influences your mind and body
- help you to work through the layers of emotions and feelings inside of you
- reveal the root of a feeling, which may be covered in layers to be released
- heal and release the painful emotions and feelings that are stuck inside you

I recommend that you treat the dictionary as a sacred, private space where you can sit with your emotions and feelings, where you can greet your emotions and feelings rather than bury, deny, dismiss, suppress, oppress or fight them.

I have used the Dictionary of Feelings myself over the last 12 months. It has changed my life. It has empowered me. I am hoping it can help you too.

Part 2: How to work successfully with your whole self
will help you to apply all the information you have read in Part 1
into practical steps so you can work successfully with your mental,
emotional, physical, spiritual and whole self.

In this part you will take the final step:

Step 4: To work _with_ yourself and not _against_ yourself

You will do this through:
   Observation: To carefully look at what is happening to you
   Introspection: To analyse and examine your whole self
   Exercises: Activities or tasks to act on so you can make
a change
   Practises: A new way to try something, and then repeat it
so it becomes part of your every day
   Check In: To turn inwards and check in with yourself,
mentally, emotionally, physically and spiritually

"The work before the work"

It is also important for you to know that this guide is not a one-
time read. It is a guide that you will need to go back to again
and again – at different times in your life, something inside of
you will call you, tell you to reach for what you need, and guide
you towards the words you need to connect to.

WHAT IS "THE WORK BEFORE THE WORK"?
In the world of psychology, when a person is struggling in life
(inside and out), and needs help to see inside their mind and

body so they can work through past emotions, thoughts and feelings, this is called inner work.

Inner work means:

- self-exploring
- self-understanding
- self-reflection
- self-healing

How do you Feel? can help you do the inner work little by little every day, or when you feel called to do so. This will hopefully enable you to take care of yourself or avoid a position where you need to seek professional help. <u>It will show you new ways to see yourself</u>, and ways to sit with and create space for the parts of yourself that you are struggling to see or connect with.

More importantly, this guide can prevent you from moving into a dark space, as you take the steps to see your whole self, inside and out. It is a guide that can point you in the right direction when you feel blocked or stuck, when you are hurting or need healing, or when you feel you are making unconscious choices and decisions each day. You can use this guide to help you make sense of yourself, or to help you to come back to the truth of yourself when you lose yourself.

The voice of this guide

This guide has been created to help <u>you</u> to see <u>your</u> whole self clearly and to work with your whole self, inside and out. As such, it is important that the voice in this guide is clean and simple to understand and contains no distracting personal stories or unnecessary facts and figures that can divert you away from the goal of this guide.

The Blank Canvas

Finally, I would like to introduce a concept that appears in this guide in selective chapters to help you see yourself clearly. It is called a Blank Canvas – a white, blank canvas is clear, pure and transparent; it is a space for you to look at yourself clearly and see your truth of your experience as you read these chapters. By using these blank canvases you can look closely at what is happening inside you – your true inner thoughts and feelings, your internal narrative.

Use the blank canvas as a space in which to make a note of your:

- emotions
- feelings

- thoughts
- opinions
- conclusions
- judgements

This is your internal narrative.

Even if you are struggling with processing your words, or are rejecting my words, still try to write the struggle down.

PART 1

HOW DO YOU FEEL?
GAINING AWARENESS

Awareness is to:

- **see:** which is to observe
- **know:** which is to recognize
- **understand:** which is to know the meaning of

To step into awareness is to move your mind into a space where you can see, know and understand what is happening to you. It is here, in this space of awareness, that you gain a chance to see yourself clearly, inside and out.

What you need to know about Part 1

Every word in Part 1 has been carefully and consciously chosen to help you become aware of yourself, inside and out, and help you see yourself as a whole. Each word has been written with a reason, a purpose and a meaning.

There is an asterisk – * – placed next to certain words. These words are further explored underneath the paragraph. I have done this to help you create space for your mind, slow down and learn to sit with and see meaning behind words.

You may sense empty space between the text in Part 1, and your sense is right. I have deliberately left gaps in places where authors usually place stories or scientific data to help the reader connect to the author, or to prove a point. Instead, I would like to help you create space in your mind so you can see yourself, and try to see beyond the words I am writing. Too many words will not help that process.

I have deliberately magnified Part 1; it is made to appear bigger than it needs to be. Part 1 is meant to help you to create space in your mind so you can step into a space of awareness. It is meant to help you see parts of yourself you cannot see, or have not had a chance to see or understand. It is meant to help you see what is important.

1
HOW DO YOU FEEL?
ALL PARTS AS A WHOLE

Step 1: Awareness: to see, to know, to understand all parts of you – as a whole.

The first step you need to take is to go back to basics and become aware of all the individual parts of "who you are", which come together to create the "whole" you. When you see your whole self clearly, you will see yourself holistically so you can better connect and interconnect, intertwine and link yourself to others – and to life as a whole.

The "ten parts" of you

There are ten parts that contribute to who you are and how you feel. They play a significant role in shaping, moulding and creating every part of your being. They bring you into existence and help you to move through life; they help you develop and grow and evolve into a person, a character and a human being.

These ten parts help you move through life and offer you human experiences as you make your way through your journey.

These ten parts are your power and guide – if you are aware of them. If you can see them, know them, understand them, then you will connect to them and work with them. Together, you will move through your life experiences successfully, allowing space and room for your entire being to evolve.

However, if you remain unaware of these ten parts – if you ignore, dismiss, bury, suppress, fight them – they can get stuck inside of you. This will cause struggle and resistance within you, and can keep you stuck in a cycle of repeating patterns that no longer serve you well in your life.

Why I wrote this chapter

If you find yourself stuck or struggling mentally, emotionally, physically or spiritually, you may find yourself searching for help. There are many self-help books available that give advice on how you can help yourself "change" your mindset, "change" your thoughts, "change" your feelings, "change" your behaviour. But how can you change these parts if you have not created the time and space to become fully aware of them – of what they are, of what they do, of what they mean, and of how they work with you?

You need to first of all see, know and understand:

1. What is the **mind**?
2. What is the **body**?
3. What is the **spirit**?
4. What are **instincts**?
5. What are **senses**?
6. What are **emotions**?
7. What are **feelings**?
8. What are **thoughts**?

9. What are **reactions**?
10. What are **behaviours**?

After reading about each part, take a moment to pause and see if you can connect to that part of you, inside and out.

1 – MIND
The mind is the part of you that is aware of your inner and outer world by *observing, *perceiving, thinking and *feeling.

Your mind is:
Conscious: Fully aware and responds to your daily life and environment
Subconscious: Not fully aware, but stores your life experiences, movements, memories, teachings, beliefs, skills, habits, patterns, reactions, actions and behaviours
Unconscious: Unaware of what is happening, yet automatically responds

*Observing: Seeing it as it is
*Perceiving: Making sense of your experiences through your senses
*Feeling: Connecting to energy or emotion

2 – BODY
Your body is the part of you that is *physical, and which is seen on the outside by others and is felt on the inside by you. Your body has an internal system in place that helps you stay alive.

Your body is:

Inside: The internal components such as brain, spine, organs; the internal systems such as nervous system, skeletal, muscular, cardiovascular, lymphatic, respiratory, digestive, urinary, reproductive and endocrine. All of these can be affected by instincts, emotions, feelings, sensations, memories and thoughts.

Outside: Your physical appearance – from the shape of your nose to the colour of your skin, the size of your feet, to the texture of your hair and everything in between.

*Physical: Relating to the physical world, the one that you can see

3 – SPIRIT

Your spirit is the part of you that is unseen, but which brings you to life, connects you to life and helps you move through life.

Your spirit is ***infinite**; it transcends beyond space and time and connects you to the sacred energy of life, which is an energy that connects to you *all* of life and all of humankind. When you leave this life, your spirit will leave your physical body behind.

*Infinite: Limitless or endless in space and time

4 – INSTINCTS

Your instincts are the part of you that moves beyond thinking and feeling.

Your instincts are **instinctive** – they will react instantly without any thought, thinking, feeling or reason. Your instincts are heavily tied to human nature and will give you the power to *connect, *protect and *survive.

*Connect: Bring together
*Protect: Keep safe from harm
*Survive: To exist

5 – SENSES
Your senses are the part of you that *identifies and explores life,
your life experiences and the world you live in.

Your senses are:
Sight
Sound
Smell
Taste
Touch

Your senses see, hear, smell, taste and feel, helping you to
identify the world around you by working with the mind and
body. It is through your senses that you *perceive; it is through
your senses you create a *perception in your mind.

*Identify: To recognize and understand
*Perceive: To become aware and conscious
*Perception: The way something is regarded and understood

6 – EMOTIONS
Your emotions are the part of you that feels an experience in
your mind – they form your *mental state.

As your mind becomes aware of your inner and outer worlds,
an *energy will stir. This energy will start in your mind and
channel itself toward your body. The energy in motion is known
as emotion. There will be many emotions that pass through the

mind and body, and they place the mind and body into three types of state.

Your emotional states are:
Positive: Feel good in the mind
Neutral: Feel okay in the mind
Negative: Feel bad in the mind

*Energy: Electrical impulses and magnetic waves that vibrate through your brain and body
*Mental state: A condition your mind is in

7 – FEELINGS
Your feelings are the part of you that feels an experience in your body through ***sensations** – they form your *physical state.

The brain and the central nervous system will be the first parts of the body that detect the energy in motion. This energy will move through the body as a sensation. The sensation will form into a feeling. This feeling will rise in your whole body or in separate parts of your body, and will place your body in three states.

The three feeling states are:
Positive: Feel good
Neutral: Feel neutral
Negative: Feel bad

*Physical state: A condition your body is in
*Sensation: A physical feeling resulting from contact with the body

8 – THOUGHTS

Your thoughts are the part of you that comes from the words formed in your mind as you feel and experience life.

Your thoughts are *created to help you:
-**make sense** of what you are experiencing
-**think** for yourself and make judgements and decisions
-**gain a** *perspective** on what you are experiencing

*Create: To bring into existence
*Perspective: The view of how you see something

9 – REACTIONS

Your reactions are the part of you that responds to energy, emotions, feelings, thoughts, sensations and vibrations.

Your reactions are the way your mind and body respond to what you are feeling and experiencing inside and outside of you.

If you become aware that you are experiencing a reaction, take a moment to create space for yourself and consider fully what your mind and body are doing. In that space of awareness you can if you feel you need to create a change in your reaction.

10 – BEHAVIOURS

Your behaviours are the part of you that determines how you act towards yourself or another.

Your behaviours are both:
Instinctive: Natural, not learned or influenced, and
Learned: Influenced, taught or copied
Your behaviours will turn into:

Habits: A repeated action, or
Patterns: A recurring way of acting

Seeing your ten parts

CREATION
These ten parts have been brought into existence based on all that you have perceived, seen, absorbed, felt and experienced in life; they are based on all that you have been through in your mind and body and have felt in your spirit.

MOVEMENT
These ten parts have moved with you, have grown with you, have developed with you, and have tried to work with you as you have experienced life.

THE ROLES THEY PLAY INSIDE AND OUTSIDE
Your **mind** is inside: it observes, perceives, feels, thinks, connects.
Your **body** is inside and outside: it connects, feels and moves.
Your **spirit** is inside: it brings life, feels life, connects to life.
Your **instincts** are inside: they move beyond thinking and feeling, they connect.
Your **senses** are inside and outside: they see, hear, smell, taste and touch.
Your **emotions** are inside: they feel experiences in the mind as good, neutral or bad.
Your **feelings** are inside: they feel experiences in the body as good, neutral or bad.
Your **thoughts** are inside: they are words in your mind created from feelings and experiences.

Your **reactions** are inside and outside: they respond to energy, emotions, feelings, vibrations and sensations.

Your **behaviours** are outside: they are how you act, either through instinct or learning, and they turn into habits and patterns.

ARE YOU AWARE OF EACH PART OF YOU?

Are you aware of your Mind?

Are you aware of your Body?

Are you aware of your Spirit?

Are you aware of your Instincts?

Are you aware of your Senses?

Are you aware of your Emotions?

Are you aware of your Feelings?

Are you aware of your Thoughts?

Are you aware of your Reactions?

Are you aware of your Behaviours?

Working in alignment with your ten parts

If you are aware, and these ten parts are seen, known and understood by you, you will naturally place yourself in alignment with your whole self. To be aligned means to have everything in the right place.

Working in alignment with your ten parts also means you will not ignore, deny, fight with or work against them. You will place yourself in harmony – a state of agreement. And to be in alignment and in harmony means you flow: you move naturally and steadily, as if you are in a continuous stream. There is no struggle or resistance. All your parts move together, in the same direction, even through times of movement and change, even if these times are turbulent, even if life changes and the ground shifts beneath you.

Being aware of your emotions, thoughts and feelings means you can be aware of and work with your reactions, actions and behaviours.

When your ten parts are working in alignment, your:
Mind is aware, clear, clean, conscious, seen, understood.
Body is balanced, nourished, strengthened.
Spirit is connected, flowing.
Instincts are seen, understood.
Senses are connected, used.
Emotions are acknowledged, seen, understood, released.
Feelings are acknowledged, seen, understood, released.
Thoughts are flowing, passing, released.
Reactions are acknowledged, seen, understood.
Behaviours are acknowledged seen, understood.

Whole self is aligned, connected, understood, seen, complete. The result of this is that you feel seen, connected, understood, whole.

Working against your ten parts

If your ten parts are not in your awareness, and not seen, known or understood by you, they will not fully connect to you and you will be "misaligned". When you are in misalignment, it will naturally create a state of disharmony, as you will not be working with yourself, but moving in different or opposite directions. This does not create flow; rather, it creates some form of disruption, resistance or struggle, which means you will find it hard to move gracefully or effortlessly through your life experiences, especially through times of turbulence and change.

At times like these, you will:

- bury
- deny
- dismiss
- fight
- hide
- ignore
- misuse
- misidentify
- push
- reject
- suppress

parts of you, such as your emotions, thoughts and feelings. Or you may deny reactions, actions and behaviours that do not align with the truth of who you are. This can cause you to become out of balance and cause a struggle inside yourself. You will not feel whole, as you will want to be seen, known or understood by others, but you will not be taking the time and space to see, know and understand yourself. What you need is not outside yourself, it is inside.

If this is how it is for you, and you find yourself struggling to work with or working against the ten parts of you, you will be feeling the following:

Mind is distorted, distracted, influenced, overloaded, unconscious.

Body is imbalanced, neglected, misused, mistreated.

Spirit is blocked, denied, suppressed, stuck.

Instincts are disconnected, blocked.

Senses are blocked, misused, mistreated.

Emotions are buried, dismissed, ignored, misunderstood, misused.

Feelings are buried, dismissed, ignored, misunderstood, misused.

Thoughts are abnormal, intrusive, obsessive, repeated, unreleased.

Reactions are unacknowledged, impulsive, reckless.

Behaviours are aggressive, defensive, denied, destructive, intransigent.

Whole self is misaligned, disconnected, misunderstood, unseen, unwhole.

The result is that you will not feel seen, understood, connected, whole.

Experiencing the ten parts – how do you feel?

The way that you experience these ten parts is dependent on how you feel inside your mind and body and on what you are experiencing in your external life.

Do you feel good, or do you feel bad?

If you feel good already, then it is easier for you to be in alignment and harmony; it is easier for you to agree with and work with the ten parts of you. When you feel good, you feel safe and you trust, so it is easier for you to accept, acknowledge and surrender to all parts of yourself and to your entire being.

However, if you feel bad, it is harder for you to be in alignment and in harmony. It is harder for you to accept, acknowledge and trust what is happening to you. It is harder for you to surrender to all parts of you and surrender to your entire being. You may be struggling to understand yourself, or see clearly, or be hurting and in pain, and so you do not trust.

Other things to be aware of . . .

BE AWARE OF THE NATURE OF LIFE

Life moves and evolves and changes, and as this happens, so can you. If you are struggling with parts of yourself or working against parts of yourself... or you feel stuck or blocked in any way – it does not have to stay this way. Life moves, and so can you. You can move through what you are experiencing inside of you and outside of you. Remembering the nature of life helps you to let go – to surrender and gracefully move through what you need to, without holding on too tight or struggling too much.

BE AWARE OF THE CORE OF YOU

Deep down, in the centre of your being, is your core, which is central to your whole existence. This core is your natural state of being. It is the part of you that connects you to life, and connects you to the ten parts of who you are. The core is the part of you that will stay as it is no matter what you are experiencing and going through. It is the truth of who you are in your life, regardless of the stage or phase you are in or of any change you are going through. If you feel disconnected from your true self because of your life experiences, your core is the part of you that will bring you back to the centre of who you are and give you a chance to see all parts of you. Be aware of your core.

BE AWARE OF THE PAST AND PRESENT

Your emotions, feelings and thoughts drive your reactions, actions and behaviours in life. If you are unaware that your past can sometimes merge with the present, or if you do not know how to separate your past emotions, feelings and thoughts from your present self, you will unconsciously and automatically react to what is happening to you in the present moment in a way that is influenced by past experience. The past can influence and contaminate your present mind and body, and affect your way of thinking and feeling, your reactions, actions and behaviours, and keep you stuck. You will not be reacting from a pure space, and this can prevent you from moving through your experiences successfully, and stop you from evolving or growing. This is misalignment.

BE AWARE OF WHO YOU ARE AND WHERE YOU ARE GOING

Each moment of your life is an opportunity to create space for yourself, and to choose whether to stay the same or make changes in your life. How you choose to work with yourself as a whole, and how you work with all the different parts of you can lead you in to two different directions and on to two very different paths.

THE PATH OF EMPOWERMENT

The path of **empowerment** will raise your mind and body to a higher level, and help you evolve into the highest version of your whole self as you "**work with**" all the parts of who you are. On this path you will be aware of each part of you that you are experiencing and feeling and react and act and behave in ways that align with your true self as a whole. You will be aware of who you are and who you want to be, and be aware and conscious of the life you want to lead.

If you feel bad, uncomfortable, or are suffering or in pain when you are on the path of empowerment, you will not add to your hurt and pain by reacting or acting in ways that create further destruction to yourself or to others in life. You will learn to move through what you are going through with power and grace, and learn to see, know and understand all parts of yourself. You will be able to trust yourself so you can work with or through the parts of you that feel bad in a successful way.

The path of empowerment will help you grow and develop and evolve to connect to yourself and to others in life and to life as a whole. This way of being – connection, unity and wholeness – will empower you.

THE PATH OF DESTRUCTION

The path of **destruction** will place your mind and body on a lower vibration as you struggle to work with yourself and your experiences. This struggle will lead you away from the path of empowerment, as you will not know how to work with your truth. You will unconsciously react and behave in ways that are in misalignment with who you are as a whole.

If you have had a bad experience, feel bad or uncomfortable, or are experiencing suffering or pain while on the path to destruction, you will choose to bury, deny, dismiss, ignore or reject parts of yourself, and you will keep reacting and behaving from this place of suffering and pain. This can cause you to be stuck, and can block you from parts of yourself and from moving forward in life. As you work against yourself, it will feel as if life is against you. You will unconsciously add to your hurt and create further pain and suffering to yourself and others in life. This path leads to an internal or external war, and causes disconnection, division and polarization.

Finally...

BE AWARE OF ALL TEN PARTS, INSIDE AND OUT

It is incredibly important to take the time to understand all the ten parts that connect within you to make you whole. They are you, they create you, they are with you each and every day. You cannot escape them. This is why you need to take that first step to see your whole self as clearly as you can. You, and all the parts of who you are in life, are a creation.

Your mind

Your body

Your spirit

Your senses,

Your emotions

Your feelings

Your thoughts

Your instincts

Your reactions

Your behaviours ...

... have all come into being based on your life experience, your life views, your perspectives, your conditioning and your teachings and learnings.

Can you answer:

Who am I?

How did I create myself into being?

How did I become who I am today?

THE BLANK CANVAS

Use the empty space below to note down what this chapter has made you think about and how it has made you feel.

Did you experience any emotions or feelings?

Did you form any new or surprising thoughts or opinions?

Did you come to any conclusions or judgements?

Use the space below to expose, truthfully and clearly, your internal narrative – make it seen.

2
HOW DO YOU FEEL?
AS YOURSELF – INSIDE AND OUT

Step 2: Awareness: to see, to know, to understand yourself – inside and out.

The second step is for you to be aware of yourself inside and out – to be aware of how you have created yourself into existence based on your life experiences and your life journey.

Your life journey

What I mean when I say "life experiences" and "life journey" is _all_ that you have been through in your life – mentally, emotionally, physically and spiritually. It is your entire self, in your past, in your present _and_ your future self. It is you as a new-born – a pure human being; it is you as a toddler and infant – learning all the time; it is you as a teenager and an adult – absorbing, seeing, perceiving, feeling. It is all that you have experienced, and how you experienced it given your situation, your views at that particular time in your life. It is every move, every sensation, every vibration, every emotion, every feeling, every thought, every reaction that has turned into an action, a behaviour or some form of physical creation. It is all that has impacted you or influenced you or changed you or shaped you, and moulded you and turned you into who _you_ are today.

Why did I write this chapter?

IF YOU ARE STUCK

When you find yourself stuck in life, and are searching for help to become unstuck, move forward or change your ways, you might be advised by guides, teachers or professionals to release old emotions or beliefs, or old opinions or habits, that no longer serve you. You might feel the need or want to change your perception or perspective. But before you can make these changes, you need to figure out where or why you are stuck or struggling inside of you and outside of you.

This chapter will help you to:

- Be aware of yourself: inside and out
- See yourself: Who are you?
- Know yourself: What do you do when you do it?
- Understand yourself: Why do you do what you do?

It will help you understand how your:

- habits
- patterns
- opinions
- judgements

- conclusions
- beliefs ...

... are created and formed.

It will help you see, know and understand how each moment of your life has served to create the whole of you, inside and out. Once you can see this, and be aware of this, it will be easier for you to see and pinpoint where or why you are getting stuck or blocked. It will be easier for you to see how patterns and habits are formed and why you struggle to let go of patterns that do not serve you. Importantly, through gaining this knowledge and understanding, you will create a space in which you can change yourself.

Stages of life

Birth: Birth is the beginning of your existence.

You are born into a new world.

You transition from your mother's womb into a new world, an unknown environment.

Body: The physical part of you

Your body – the physical part of you that is felt and seen – enters the world, and with it are your mind, senses, instincts and spirit.

Change:
In this new, unfamiliar environment you are surrounded by unfamiliarity and change.

Movement:

With change, there is movement. There is movement outside of you and inside of you.

The world is moving around you. This is the movement of life.

Energy:

With life, there is energy – magnetic waves that vibrate through mind and body. This energy flows through your mind and body. Energy moves through life and connects life with other life.

It is energy that creates emotions, feelings and states.

Emotions and Feelings:

An energy will stir in your mind; it will channel its way from the mind toward your body.

The energy will turn into a sensation, which will turn into a feeling.

Feelings are a condition your body is in, and are experienced as...

- **Positive:** I am feeling good
- **Neutral:** I am feeling okay
- **Negative:** I am feeling bad

A State of Mind and Being:

States are a condition your mind and body are in, and are experienced as . . .

Positive: You are enjoying the experience

Neutral: You are neutral to the experience

Negative: You are not enjoying the experience

Moments:

A moment is an exact point in time you are experiencing life.

These positive, neutral, negative states you are experiencing are fleeting: they should only last for a very short time, passing through your mind and body in moments.

Time: A continued progression of existence

As your mind and your body move through moments of your life, the time you are in will be measured by seconds, minutes, hours and days. The first day of your life is experienced in 24 hours. You will absorb the surroundings and feel the movement of life. You will feel movement in the form of breath energy and vibrations. You will feel movement with emotions, feelings and sensations.

Life:

The **positive, neutral** or **negative state** is a condition your mind and body is in at the exact **moment** you have a life experience. When you are in the present moment, you absorb your surroundings and feel the movement. You feel the movement of life through emotions, feelings and sensations, which come into the present, and then go into the past, leaving you ready to experience the future – the cycle of **life.**

Your mind, body and spirit are now ready to experience a new day.

This is the power of life. You will be in it and experience it . . . and then it moves on.

There is a future. It is waiting for you. And it will come in time with the movement of your life.

Your growth:

DEVELOPMENT STAGES

Over the years of your life you will experience changes in your mind and body as you develop and grow. These stages are infancy, childhood, adolescence, early adulthood, middle age, old age.

Phases:

If your mind or body is not ready to enter the next development stage of your life it will go through a phase – the step from one stage to another – during which your mind and body catch up with the new changes in your life.

Life experiences: knowledge gained through living

As your mind and body start to move forward in life, you will experience places and spaces.

Places

These are . . .

Environments: An environment is the surroundings and conditions that you are in.

And . . .

Spaces: an unoccupied area of life you are in.

These **spaces** are filled by:

- **events:** something that happens in your life that may be expected or unexpected
- **circumstances:** an event or fact that causes something to happen
- **situations:** a set of circumstances in which you find yourself, either alone or with others
- **outcomes:** the way something turns out, which might be expected or unexpected

In these places and spaces your mind and body will be placed in a...

Position: a place where you are

From the position of your mind and body, you will have a...

Viewpoint: a position that is giving you a good view

From this viewpoint, your mind and body will have a...

View: the ability to see something from a particular place

From this view, your **mind** will create a...

Perception: using all senses to understand and interpret what you experience

From this **perception** you will gain a...

Perspective: a particular way of viewing something; a point of view

And from this **perception, perspective** and **point of view** you will experience...

Emotions: An experience in your mind that moves your body into a state

Feelings: An experience or sensation or vibration in your body

On

The INSIDE: The inside world that you live in and experience

In

The UNSEEN: The stirring, of energy emotions, feelings, thoughts, sensations, on the inside of you

There are many emotions and feelings that will pass through your mind and body, every second of your day, they are part of human nature, and essential to survival.

It is from your emotions and feelings you will have a . . .

Reaction: a response to what is happening, from energy, emotions, sensations.
The reaction you will have is going to be either:
Mental: related to your mind (inside of your mind)

OR

Physical: related to your body (inside of your body, outside of your body)

This is when your mind will start to form what you are experiencing into:

Words: communication

These words will turn into:

Thoughts: an idea or opinion that is forming in your mind

Opinions: the way you see it based on your position and viewpoint

Conclusions: a decision reached; a result – how it is

Judgements: coming to a conclusion – this is how it is

Beliefs: an acceptance of how it is–it exists, it is true.

Your experience will either stay inside of you or be released outside of you

via

Expression: the action of emotions, feelings, thoughts, stirring inside of you

and

Language: A verbal and non-verbal expression of communication

Language will be:

Verbal: spoken communication

Body: unspoken, spoken through the body

This language will be turned into:

Behaviour: how you act

Natural behaviour comes from within; it is who you are and how you are naturally. When you feel aligned and connected to your life, your behaviour will be natural.

Learned behaviour is what has been taught to you or shown to you by others. It is how you think you should be, but it is not natural for you. Learned behaviour can be misaligned and disconnected from your truth.

Masked behaviour is created to conceal (hide) your true feelings, often from fear. It is misaligned and disconnected from large parts of your truth.

Your behaviour, if repeated, will turn into:

Habits: a repeated act
In an automatic way, your **habits** will turn into . . .

Patterns: a repeated way of being
It is your habits, patterns and behaviour that will start to shape your character. Your character will be part of your personality, your personality is what creates a unique version of yourself.

THIS IS YOU

The way that you experience yourself and your life is through a . . .
Life Lens: the lens through which you look at life
It is through your lens that you will have a . . .

Life View: your unique perception of life
This **life view** will give you a . . .

World View: your perception of the world
Your character and personality is what makes you individual and human. Your mental, emotional, physical and spiritual experiences – the person you were, are and will be – form your mind, body and spirit as a whole.

This is what gives you a human life and a human experience.

What do you need to be aware of?

THE WORK: This is where the work needs to start.

YOUR CREATION

Every reaction and action is part of the process of bringing you into existence. As your mind and body start to shape, mould and form into who you are – based on all that you have seen, and all that you have perceived; based on the environments, events, circumstances, situations you have been exposed to; on every energy, emotion, feeling, thought and sensation that you have ever felt; and on every position and viewpoint you have ever held – the true you will come into existence.

YOUR STORAGE

There is space available inside of you for storing the future you. As you start forming into you, your mind will store all of your life experiences in the subconscious. It will store your version of those life events in the form of memories, energy, vibrations, emotions and feelings, some which will be unprocessed. It also stores thoughts, opinions, conclusions, judgements and beliefs; and the way you react and act, and your behaviours, habits and patterns.

RESURFACE

This storage is all the parts that you have been and are, based on your life and what you feel and are taught. They are there inside you, and as life starts to move forward some of those parts will **resurface**. What might resurface could include energy, emotions, feelings, memories, thoughts, beliefs, opinions, and wounds that were created inside of you at a previous time in your life.

REPLAY

If you happen to find yourself in a similar <u>place</u> or <u>space</u> as in the past, your brain will compare current and past experiences. It may **replay** old emotions, thoughts, opinions, beliefs or feelings back to you. It may replay the same words, opinions, conclusions or judgements as if they exist in the present time.

This happens in order to help <u>you remember that you have experienced this before</u>, and enable you to <u>deal with the situation and react in the same way or in a different way as is appropriate. This replay allows you to make a choice and evolve as a person.</u>

REPEAT

When external events are repeated, it may feel strange – as if you are experiencing the same space and place, the same position in life again. This can influence how you feel in the present moment and cause mixed feelings. This can cause old wounds to resurface and make you realize that they need to be seen in order to heal.

OLD WOUNDS

Old wounds are hurt and pain caused by past events – negative emotions that have been pushed aside or buried deep inside the mind and body.

The cause of the wounds felt bad at the time you experienced them, and they have not had a chance to be healed and released; they have lain dormant, beneath other feelings. When these negative feelings start to awaken, it will feel like an old wound is opening up inside of you, and this will cause double the amount of pain.

Recurring experiences

This will feel like a recurring experience, as if life is repeating the same bad events again. You will start to feel unsettled, uncomfortable and bad on the inside. Because you will feel as if life has placed you into the same place and position again, you may repeat (consciously or unconsciously) your past reactions. This may not serve you well if you are reacting from unprocessed emotions or feelings, or if you are stuck in layers of negative emotional states.

What happens if you are unaware?

If you choose not to "see" yourself, if you choose not to "know" yourself, if you choose not to "understand" yourself, you can end up **repeating old reactions**. You may unconsciously react or act in the same way as you did in the past, or naturally move back into your old habits as it feels easier than trying to change.

Or you can end up **repeating old ways** – moving back to a former practice, condition, judgement, belief.

This means you are **stuck**, as if you are in a cycle or a circle. This will cause your feelings to be influenced or contaminated with emotions, feelings and thoughts from the past, and you will unconsciously keep recreating old emotions, feelings, thoughts, judgements, opinions and beliefs.

Your old wounds, which are stored in your subconscious, will hurt you again and again when they resurface; this will cause you to experience double the emotional pain inside of you, one layer over another. This will cause you to struggle with yourself, inside and out, and to have your life lens clouded by trapped, past emotions rather than being clear in the pure, present moment.

A distorted life view

Being unaware means you can have a **distorted life view**. Your perception of life might have been pulled and twisted out of shape based on how you feel. The way you view your life is based on how you feel about life. If you feel positive, you have an optimistic view; if you feel neutral you will have a clear view; if you feel negative, you will have a pessimistic view.

The influence of your distorted life view will seep into your life outside, and distort your world view. And this influence will seep into your physical life.

Be aware of the unseen

In the unseen, or the space in between, there is a stirring of energy and emotions and feelings, which turn into words, thoughts, opinions and judgements on the inside of you.

This is a lonely, dark space where every move, every sensation, every vibration, every emotion, every feeling, every thought, every reaction is felt and stored, from past to present. It is here that you may find it hard to find the right words to connect with and explain. It is here where you bury, dismiss, fight, hide, ignore, misuse, misidentify, reject and suppress all that you are seeing, experiencing and feeling inside of you.

Be aware of negative emotions and feelings and double pain

If you do not work with your negative emotions and feelings or the old painful emotions and feelings that rise inside you, you will end up on a path of internal struggle and double pain. When you feel bad, additional layers of emotions will be repeatedly added each time the negative emotions resurface, as they will be trying to help you make it through the pain. If you do not try to see, know and understand this, you will suffer unnecessarily by (unconsciously or consciously) repeating old, negative habits or behaviours, or reacting in negative ways or patterns that do not serve you.

The only way to empower yourself is to work with the unseen parts of you, especially the emotions, the feelings, that are inside of you. If you can clearly see your emotions and feelings, and know and understand what each one means, especially the ones that are hurting you, or keeping you stuck and blocked and preventing you from evolving, you will be able to work with the parts of yourself that can help you to grow and evolve and align. By doing this you will be on the path to empowerment of your whole self.

This is why it is vitally important that you are deeply aware of who you are, and how you feel – why it is vitally important that you understand all the ten parts that create you into who you are. By being aware of what is happening inside, you can ensure that your emotions and feelings move through your mind and body and do not get stuck or stored in your subconscious.

THE BLANK CANVAS

Use the empty space below to note down what this chapter has made you think about and how it has made you feel.

Did you experience any emotions or feelings?

Did you form any new or surprising thoughts or opinions?

Did you come to any conclusions or judgements?

Use the space below to expose, truthfully and clearly, your internal narrative – make it seen.

3
DICTIONARY OF FEELINGS: INTRODUCTION

Step 3: Awareness: to see, to know, to understand your emotions and feelings.

The third step you need to take is for you to be aware of – see, know, understand – each emotion and feeling that passes through your mind and body as you experience life in real time. The purpose of emotions and feelings is to:

- **connect:** join together, bind and unite
- **protect:** keep safe from harm and danger
- **drive:** to move in the direction of

You are not alone

No one on this earth is immune to emotions and feelings, or the pain and suffering and discomfort of negative emotions and feelings that pass through the mind and body. Feelings and emotions are part of the human experience. It is part of human life.

HOW DO YOU FEEL IN YOUR MIND AND BODY?

However, you are alone in your own mind and body. Only you will know how it feels as you experience life from your position or point of view, and as you experience specific events and circumstances and situations. Only you can truly know what emotion and feeling is passing through you at the present moment, and whether how you feel is based purely on the present moment or if it is influenced by a past experience.

The Dictionary of Feelings

The Dictionary of Feelings contains over 140 emotions and feelings that can help you to be aware of what is happening to you inside your mind and body. It can help you step into awareness and see and know and understand what each emotion and feeling means.

The dictionary is split into three parts:

Part 1: **Positive** – feels good
Part 2: **Neutral** – feels neutral
Part 3: **Negative** – feels bad

The words in each part relate to the emotions and feelings that impact or describe your mental and physical states.

A STATE OF MIND AND BEING
Each emotion and feeling will be described as a state of mind and being. The reason for this is that when your mind and body feel an emotion or feeling, and it passes through your mind and body, your mind and body will move into a state and out

of a state. As this is an holistic guide, you should be aware that what you experience in your mind, mentally, impacts you emotionally and also impacts you physically and spiritually. It is all connected.

DICTIONARY FORMAT

Each word in the dictionary is formatted as follows:

Meaning: What the emotion and feeling mean

Purpose: How the emotion and feeling are trying to help you

Feeling: Examples of other emotions and feelings that feel the same way – **the examples**

What happens to the body? How your body will be impacted

> **Warning**: it is important you are aware of this. The mind and body process life and emotions in different ways. Take the information here as an example of how your body could react. It is also important to be aware that new studies in this field are constantly happening, and the science is being updated all the time.

Inside: How it feels inside of the mind and body

Outside: How it impacts you outside of the body

Reaction: How you may react to what you are feeling on the inside

Root: The leading emotion that drives all the other – the base

THE ROOT

The roots are emotions that lie at the base of all the other emotions and feelings. There are four emotions that have been carefully chosen as roots; they are pure and are easy to understand. These four roots are heavily tied to your human instincts, and are the first emotions to connect and protect you in life. They are the first emotions (in my view) that will lead you into a positive or negative state and out of a positive or negative state. It is important, as you work with yourself, that you are able to work through the layers of emotions you feel inside of you, but more importantly, it is very important you reveal the root. Why is this? If the root of how you feel is revealed, it can heal you; it can help you to see your truth; it can change and transform and move your entire being and lead you back to you. The root of how you feel holds a power and vibration that you should be aware of.

HOW TO USE THE DICTIONARY?

When an emotion or feeling stirs or rises in your mind or in your body, take some time to consider how it is making you feel – good, neutral or bad – and then head to the relevant chapter: positive, neutral or negative.

In the chosen chapter, search for the name of the emotion or feeling. **Sit with the word** and see if its meaning and purpose make sense to you and connect with you. Allow yourself time and space to sit with the truth of how you feel in mind and body, and allow yourself time and space to be aware of emotions and feelings.

Say the words: *I feel... .* This helps you to move what is happening inside of you, in the dark, outside of you, into the daylight.

If the word and its meaning and purpose do connect with you, you have now stepped into awareness.

Allow the emotion to pass through you.

Do not hold on tight to it; rather just feel it, acknowledge it, accept it and allow the truth of how you feel to pass through you.

If the word you have chosen does not make sense to you, then look through the chapter for an alternative word that might connect better with you. Continue to do this until you reach the right word.

BE AWARE OF LAYERS

Emotions and feelings are not linear; they do not neatly progress from one stage to another. Your emotions and feelings move in cycles or circles, and can mix from past to present, or overlap one another or layer themselves on top of one another. This is especially true if your mind is not in a pure or present state; if your mind is always moving back and forth between past and present, your emotions and feelings will layer themselves.

Be aware of the emotional layers each time you feel an emotion or feeling, each time your mind and body is pushed into a state. Use the dictionary to help you work through the layers and reveal the root, so you can see the truth.

(Note: Chapters 1 and 2 will also help you to go back to basics and help you understand how thoughts, beliefs, opinions, judgements and conclusions are created, and how your emotions start to move inside of you. Being aware of this will help you to be still, and to see yourself.)

BE AWARE OF CIRCLES OR CYCLES

Circles are emotions and feelings that bring you back to the same place.

Cycles are emotions and feelings that keep repeating in the same way, and feel as if they form a circle.

As you start to move through each stage and phase of your life, your emotions and feelings will move through your mind and body. If these emotions and feelings start to feel like they are in a circle or a cycle of energy – whether it's **Positive, Neutral** or **Negative** energy – they will not be clean; rather they will be mixed up and contaminated.

How long you stay in each emotional circle or cycle will depend on how you choose to work with your emotions and feelings, and if you are aware this is happening to you.

BE AWARE OF HOW YOU WORK WITH YOUR EMOTIONS AND FEELINGS

Do you work with or do you work against your emotions and feelings?

If you work with then you will be aware, accept and acknowledge them. You will be in alignment, agreement and harmony.

If you work against then you will bury, dismiss, ignore, reject, suppress and repress them. You will be in misalignment, opposition, disagreement and disharmony.

As you work with the Dictionary of Feelings, start to see yourself and how you work with your emotions and feelings. I am aware that emotions and feelings are fleeting and pass through the mind and body very quickly. However, it is important you can clearly see the emotion or feeling that you are experiencing. To do this, you need space and to learn to see them; take time to sit with them and see them, to remember them. The only way to do this, is to magnify each one.

4
DICTIONARY OF FEELINGS – POSITIVE

What does positive mean?

Positive states are here to help you:

- live your life
- enjoy your life
- experience life
- be connected
- stay connected
- lead a fulfilling life
- improve wellbeing
- increase awareness
- increase attention and memory
- connect you to the energy of life

Positive states move from your mind toward your body and activate the reward system in your brain. This activation helps you to feel good about what you are experiencing in your mind and body, and when you start to feel good about what you are experiencing, you start to feel good about what is happening to you in that moment.

When your mind and body have entered into a positive state, this means you are experiencing a positive moment, event, circumstance, situation or outcome. This stirs a positive energy, emotion and feeling, and your mind shifts your body into a positive state. You will be seeing life through on optimistic lens.

Positive feelings can range from mild to very strong, and your vibration or mood can range from medium to very high. The autonomic nervous system, which regulates your breathing, heartbeat and digestion, is activated by positive emotions.

The root

There are two natural states that lie at the root of positive states:

- joy
- unconditional love

They are always with you, waiting to reveal themselves to you. They lie waiting for you beneath all your life experiences. When you are ready to feel good again, these two positive emotions will naturally unveil themselves to you and your mind, and your body will feel connected to life and the joy of life and the love of life again.

JOY
Meaning: A state of mind and being that helps you to connect to life and connect to the feeling of being alive.
Purpose: To help you to feel the enjoyment of life and to connect with and feel the joy of your life experiences and also to help guide you to what brings you true joy in life.

Feeling: Joy.

WHAT HAPPENS TO THE BODY?

Inside: The brain chemical dopamine, which is responsible for pleasure and reward, is released. The brain chemical serotonin, which is responsible for balancing mood and boosting wellbeing, is released. The brain chemical oxytocin, which is responsible for emotional responses and social bonding, is released. Endorphins that are responsible for boosting pleasure are released. The circulatory system, which pumps oxygen into your heart and lungs and circulates blood through the body, is boosted. The immune system, which is responsible for defence and protecting your body, is regulated and boosted.

Outside: Body relaxes, pupils dilate, eyes brighten, skin glows.

Reaction: To be (exist without resistance), to enjoy, to play, to relax, to take pleasure.

Power: To connect to life.

Vibration: High.

UNCONDITIONAL LOVE

Meaning: A state of mind and being that is connected to a love so powerful and pure and deep without expecting anything in return.

Purpose: To help you to connect to a pure love; to help you to see beyond beliefs, behaviours, emotions, feelings, judgements, thoughts, opinions, reactions, viewpoints.

Feeling: Unconditional love.

WHAT HAPPENS TO THE BODY?

Inside: The brain chemical dopamine, which is responsible for pleasure and reward, is activated. The brain chemical oxytocin, which is responsible for emotional responses and social bonding, is released. Phenylethylamine (PEA), which is an endorphin responsible for energy, alertness and heightened senses and stimulation, is released into the bloodstream. The circulation system, which is responsible for circulating blood, nutrients and cells to all of the body, is boosted. The endocrine system, which is responsible for stimulating glands and increasing oxygen and glucose into the bloodstream, is activated. Heart rate increases. Rapid breathing. Blood circulation speeds up.

Outside: Pupils dilate, eyes brighten, skin glows, body surrenders (stops resisting).

Reaction: To accept and receive embrace.

Power: To bind, to connect, to unite.

Vibration: Extremely high.

The layers

AMAZEMENT

Meaning: A state of mind and being that makes you aware that you are experiencing something out of the ordinary.

Purpose: To help you shift out of your ordinary state and experience new things.

Feeling: Awe, surprise, wonder

WHAT HAPPENS TO THE BODY?

Inside: The brain stimulates the hippocampus, which is the part of your brain responsible for memories and learning. The brain chemical dopamine, which is responsible for pleasure and reward, is released. The brain chemical serotonin, which is responsible for wellbeing, is released. Endorphins that are responsible for boosting pleasure and reducing pain are released. The circulatory system, which pumps oxygen into your heart and lungs and circulates blood through the body, is boosted. Heart rate increases. Rapid breathing.

Outside: Eyes widen, body rises, attention sharpens.

Reaction: To admire (regard with respect), to approve.

AMUSEMENT

Meaning: A state of mind and being where you find an experience, event or situation funny or entertaining.

Purpose: To help you connect with an experience.

Feeling: Cheerful, happy.

WHAT HAPPENS TO THE BODY?

Inside: The brain chemical serotonin, which is responsible for wellbeing, is released. Endorphins that are responsible for boosting pleasure and reducing pain are released. The circulatory system, which pumps oxygen into your heart and lungs and circulates blood through the body, is boosted. Heart rate increases. Rapid breathing. Muscles ease and relax.

Outside: Body relaxes, mouth forms into a smile.

Reaction: To engage (get involved).

ANTICIPATION

Meaning: A state of mind and being that makes you aware of an expected event or outcome.

Purpose: To help move you forward and help you see what may be ahead of you.

Feeling: Excitement, eagerness.

WHAT HAPPENS TO THE BODY?

Inside: The brain chemical dopamine, which is responsible for pleasure and reward and survival, is released. The circulatory system, which pumps oxygen into your heart and lungs and

circulates blood through the body, is boosted. Endorphins that are responsible for boosting pleasure and reducing pain are released into the bloodstream. Heart rate increases. Rapid breathing. Body is in eustress, which is beneficial stress.
Outside: Body moves forward.
Reaction: To prepare, to plan.

Astonishment

Meaning: A state of mind and being that makes you suddenly stop and see that the information you are receiving is way beyond what you expected to receive.

Purpose: To help you move out of your current state and shift your mind towards something you did not expect.

Feeling: Amazement, awe, surprise.

What happens to the body?

Inside: The brain stimulates the hippocampus, which is the part of your brain responsible for memories and learning. The central nervous system, which is connected to your brain and entire body, is activated. The sympathetic nervous system, responsible for releasing hormones into the bloodstream to increase alertness and energy, is activated. Adrenalin, which is responsible for increasing the heart rate, blood pressure and oxygen to the lungs, is released into the bloodstream. The circulatory system, which pumps oxygen into your heart and lungs and circulates blood through the body, is boosted. Heart rate increases. Rapid breathing.

Outside: Eyes widen, body becomes alert.

Reaction: To be startled, to jump.

AWE

Meaning: A state of mind and being that experiences something that is beautiful or sacred or unbelievable.

Purpose: To help you get out of your ordinary state and see something beautiful and sacred; to help you experience something that is far beyond your own reach and understanding.

Feeling: Amazement, surprise, wonder.

WHAT HAPPENS TO THE BODY?

Inside: The brain stimulates the hippocampus, which is the part of your brain responsible for memories and learning. Endorphins that are responsible for boosting pleasure and reducing pain are released. The circulatory system, which pumps oxygen into your heart and lungs and circulates blood through the body, is boosted. Cytokines – protein cells in your immune system – are lowered in order to promote and regulate your immune response. Heart rate increases. Breathing deepens and speeds up.

Outside: Eyes widen, body draws closer to what it is in awe of.

Reaction: To admire, to respect, to explore.

BLISS

Meaning: A state of mind and being that allows you to experience a deep state of contentment and fulfilment.

Purpose: To help you enjoy and experience the beautiful moments of your life.

Feeling: Content, happy, joy.

WHAT HAPPENS TO THE BODY?

Inside: The brain chemical dopamine, which is responsible for pleasure and reward, is released. The brain chemical serotonin, which is responsible for wellbeing, is released. Endorphins

Dictionary

that are responsible for boosting pleasure and reducing pain are released. The parasympathetic nervous system, which is responsible for rest and digestion and conserving energy, is regulated. Heartbeat slows down. Digestion increases. Breath is regulated. Muscles ease and relax.

Outside: Body is lighter, weightless.

Reaction: To flow (move in a steady, continuous stream).

CALM

Meaning: A state of mind and being where you are balanced as a whole.

Purpose: To help you remain in a calm state so you can clearly observe your surroundings and to help you to connect to all the parts of who you are.

Feeling: Peaceful, serene, tranquil.

WHAT HAPPENS TO THE BODY?

Inside: The amygdala, which is the emotional centre of the brain and the part of the brain that activates the fight-or-flight response, is decreased. The parasympathetic nervous system, which is responsible for rest and digestion and conserving energy, is regulated. Heartbeat slows down. Muscles relax.

Outside: Your body is balanced – mind, body and spirit.

Reaction: To be stable.

*Balanced: In good proportion. Mind. Body. Spirit

CAREFREE

Meaning: A state of mind and being that sets you free in the moment of your experience.

Purpose: To help you be mentally, physically, emotionally and spiritually free.

Feeling: Carefree, happy.

WHAT HAPPENS TO THE BODY?

Inside: The brain chemical oxytocin, which is responsible for social bonding, is triggered and released. The brain chemical serotonin, which is responsible for wellbeing, is released. Endorphins that are responsible for boosting pleasure and reducing pain are released. The circulatory system, which pumps oxygen into your heart and lungs and circulates blood through the body, is boosted. Heart rate increases. Rapid breathing.

Outside: Body moves with ease.

Reaction: To be free (unbound, unrestricted), to play, to find pleasure, to enjoy, to flow (move in a steady, continuous stream).

CHEERFUL

Meaning: A state of mind and being where you are happy by nature.

Purpose: To help you to connect to the brighter side of life.

Feeling: Happy, joy.

WHAT HAPPENS TO THE BODY?

Inside: The brain chemical dopamine, which is responsible for pleasure and reward, is released. The brain chemical serotonin, which is responsible for balancing mood and boosting wellbeing, is released. The brain chemical oxytocin, which is responsible for emotional responses and social bonding, is released. The circulatory system, which pumps oxygen into your heart and lungs and circulates blood through the body, is boosted.

Outside: The body is energetic and upbeat.

Reaction: To enjoy, to take pleasure.

COMFORTABLE

Meaning: A state of mind and being where your mind and body is at ease.

Purpose: To help you to be comfortable in your whole being inside and out.

Feeling: Happy, relaxed.

WHAT HAPPENS TO THE BODY?

Inside: The brain chemical dopamine, which is responsible for pleasure and reward, is released. The brain chemical serotonin, which is responsible for balancing mood and boosting wellbeing, is released. The brain chemical oxytocin, which is responsible for emotional responses and social bonding, is released. The parasympathetic nervous system, which is responsible for rest and digestion and conserving energy, is regulated. Muscles relax.

Outside: The body relaxes.

Reaction: To relax (loosen up).

COMPASSIONATE

Meaning: A state of mind and being where you feel strongly towards another person's emotions, experiences, suffering, struggle, pain, misfortune and feelings.

Purpose: To help you connect to the journey of another human being in order to understand life and others in life, and to understand yourself and humanity on a much deeper level.

Feeling: Empathy, sympathy.

WHAT HAPPENS TO THE BODY?

Inside: The visual cortex, the part of the brain that processes visual information and connects with what it is seeing or experiencing, is activated. The amygdala, the emotional centre of the part of the brain that is responsible for threat and danger and activating fight and flight, eases. The vagus nerve that connects the brain and body, and is responsible for motor information and body movement and stimulating muscles in the vocal chamber enabling open communication, is activated. The parasympathetic nervous system, which is responsible for rest and digest and conserving energy, regulates. Heartbeat slows down. Muscles ease and relax.

Outside: The body relaxes.

Reaction: To connect, to unite.

CONFIDENT

Meaning: A state of mind and being that makes you feel certain and secure in your qualities and abilities.

Purpose: To provide you with an inner knowing that you are good enough, helping you take on the external world with more energy and determination.

Feeling: Calm, connected.

WHAT HAPPENS TO THE BODY?

Inside: The prefrontal cortex, which is found in the front of your brain and is responsible for the value of decision-making, planning and behaviour, is activated. The striatus, the part of the brain that coordinates action, planning, decision-making, motivation, reward-planning and reward-perception, is activated. The brain chemical serotonin, which is responsible for balancing mood and boosting wellbeing, is released. The circulatory system, which pumps oxygen into your heart and lungs and circulates blood through the body, is boosted. The autonomic nervous system, which is responsible for your breathing, heart rate and digestion, is regulated. The immune system is boosted. Muscles ease.

Dictionary

Outside: Head held high, body posture rises tall, eyes focus.
Reaction: To believe, to connect, to trust.

CONNECTED

Meaning: A state of mind and being where you are open to connect to yourself and others, and to life itself.

Purpose: To help you connect to people and places and to help you feel an affinity (a natural likening or understanding) for life.

Feeling: Connected, confident.

WHAT HAPPENS TO THE BODY?

Inside: The brain chemical oxytocin, which is responsible for emotional responses and social bonding, is released. The brain chemical serotonin, which is responsible for balancing mood and boosting wellbeing, is released. The autonomic nervous system, which is responsible for your breathing, heart rate and digestion, is regulated. The circulatory system, which pumps oxygen into your heart and lungs and circulates blood through the body, is boosted. Muscles ease and relax. Heart rate regulates. Breathing regulates.

Outside: Body connects and relaxes.

Reaction: To accept, to embrace, to understand.

CONTENT

Meaning: A state of mind that helps you be deeply aware of what you have in your life, and you do not have a strong desire or need for it to be changed.

Purpose: To help you see clearly what you have and where you are in your life.

Feeling: Fulfilled, happy, peaceful and satisfied.

WHAT HAPPENS TO THE BODY?
Inside: The brain chemical oxytocin, which is responsible for emotional responses and social bonding, is released. The brain chemical serotonin, which is responsible for balancing mood and boosting wellbeing, is released. The nervous system, responsible for receiving information through senses and controlling regulation and communication in the body, is balanced and regulated. The immune system, which is responsible for defence and protection, is regulated. The circulatory system, which pumps oxygen into your heart and lungs and circulates blood through the body, is boosted. Muscles relax.
Outside: Body eases and relaxes.
Reaction: To accept, to appreciate.

COURAGEOUS
Meaning: A state of mind and being that gives you the strength to confront something that frightens you, despite fear, danger or disapproval.
Purpose: To help you go within and find your power and bravery in the face of fear, pain, suffering, threat or death itself.
Feeling: Confident, powerful.
WHAT HAPPENS TO THE BODY?
Inside: The anterior cingulate cortex, the front part of the brain responsible for regulating your emotions and decision-making, is activated. The amygdala, the part of the brain responsible for activating the fight-or-flight response, deactivates. The hippocampus part of the brain, which is responsible for motivation, is stimulated. The brain chemical dopamine, which is responsible for pleasure and reward, is released. The autonomic nervous system, responsible for breathing, the heart and

digestion, is balanced and regulated. The circulatory system, which pumps oxygen into your heart and lungs and circulates blood through the body, is boosted.

Outside: Body is balanced and stable.

Reaction: To be brave, to be strong, to be powerful.

DELIGHT

Meaning: A state of mind and being where you experience a sense of pure, uncomplicated pleasure.

Purpose: To help you fully enjoy a life experience.

Feeling: Happy, pleased.

WHAT HAPPENS TO THE BODY?

Inside: The brain chemical dopamine, which is responsible for pleasure and reward, is released. The brain chemical serotonin, which is responsible for balancing mood and boosting wellbeing, is released. The brain chemical oxytocin, which is responsible for emotional responses and social bonding, is released. Endorphins that are responsible for reducing pain and boosting your wellbeing are triggered and released into the bloodstream. The circulatory system, which pumps oxygen into your heart and lungs and circulates blood through the body, is boosted. The immune system, which is responsible for defence and protecting your body, is regulated and boosted. Heartbeat increases. Muscles relax.

Outside: Eyes light up, smile starts to form.

Reaction: To enjoy.

DEVOTED

Meaning: A state of mind and being where you are available to give (offer) your whole self.

Purpose: To help you to surrender (stop resisting).

Feeling: Love.

WHAT HAPPENS TO THE BODY?

Inside: The brain chemical dopamine, which is responsible for pleasure and reward, is activated. The brain chemical oxytocin, which is responsible for emotional responses and social bonding, is activated. The circulatory system, which pumps oxygen into your heart and lungs and circulates blood through the body, is regulated. The autonomic nervous system, which is responsible for breathing, heart rate and digestion, is balanced and regulated. The parasympathetic nervous system, which is responsible for rest and digestion and conserving energy, is regulated. Heartbeat slows down. Muscles relax.

Outside: Body surrenders itself to the devotion.

Reaction: To give (offer something).

ECSTATIC

Meaning: A state of mind and being that alters your state of consciousness to make you feel an intense and powerful emotion.

Purpose: To help you step out of yourself and see in a new way.

Feeling: Ecstatic, euphoric, elated, happy, joy, love, unconditional love.

WHAT HAPPENS TO THE MIND AND BODY?

Inside: The brain chemical dopamine, which is responsible for pleasure and reward, is released. The brain chemical serotonin, which is responsible for balancing mood and boosting wellbeing, is released. The brain chemical oxytocin, which is responsible for emotional responses and social bonding, is released. The circulatory system, which pumps oxygen into your heart and lungs and circulates blood through the body, is boosted. The sympathetic nervous system, responsible for releasing hormones into the bloodstream to increase alertness and energy, is activated. Adrenalin, which is responsible for increasing heart rate, raising blood pressure and increasing oxygen into lungs, is released.

Outside: Pupils dilate, body is alert.

Reaction: To act.

ELATED

Meaning: A state of mind that takes you to a very high level and vibration of joy.

Purpose: To help you be aware of what you have accomplished and achieved.

Feeling: Happy, excited, enthusiastic, satisfied.

WHAT HAPPENS TO THE BODY?

Inside: The brain chemical dopamine, which is responsible for pleasure and reward, is released. The sympathetic nervous system, which is responsible for releasing hormones into the bloodstream to increase alertness and energy, is activated. the hormone adrenalin, which is responsible for increasing the heart rate, blood pressure, oxygen to the lungs and dilating pupils, is released into the bloodstream. The circulatory system, which pumps oxygen into your heart and lungs and circulates blood through the body, is boosted. Heart rate increases. Breathing is rapid.

Outside: Body is lifted and raised.

Reaction: To be proud

EMPATHETIC

Meaning: A state of mind and being where you are fully aware and can understand and feel what another person is feeling.

Purpose: To help you be aware and understand how another person feels.

Feeling: Sympathy, compassion.
WHAT HAPPENS TO THE BODY?
Inside: The visual cortex, which is the part of the brain responsible for processing visual information, is activated. The anterior cingulate cortex, which is the part of the brain responsible for regulating emotional decision-making and attention, is activated. The brain chemical oxytocin, which is responsible for social bonding, is released. The peripheral autonomic and somatic nervous systems, responsible for communication, senses, movement and balance, are stimulated. The insula part of the nervous system, responsible for heartbeat, blood flow, breathing and digestion, is activated.
Outside: Body opens itself up to gestures and responses.
Reaction: To connect.

ENTHUSIASTIC
Meaning: A state of mind and being where you have a strong force of energy that makes you want to be fully involved in something.
Feeling: Intense, eager, enjoyment, interest, passion, approval.
WHAT HAPPENS TO THE BODY?
Inside: The brain chemical dopamine, which is responsible for pleasure and reward, is released. The sympathetic nervous system, which is responsible for releasing hormones into the bloodstream to increase alertness and energy, is activated. Adrenalin, which is responsible for increasing the heart rate, blood pressure, oxygen into the lungs and dilating pupils, is released. The circulatory system, which pumps oxygen into your heart and lungs and circulates blood through the body, is boosted.
Outside Pupils dilate, eyes widen, body is energetic.
Purpose: To help you be aware of what you're passionate about
Reaction: To engage (be involved).

Euphoric

Meaning: A state of mind and being that makes you experience an intense and very high level of joy.

Purpose: To help you be aware of an immense sense of wellbeing; to help you experience pleasure.

Feeling: Happy, elated, ecstatic.

What happens to the body?

Inside: The brain chemical dopamine, which is responsible for pleasure and reward, is released. The sympathetic nervous system, which is responsible for releasing hormones into the bloodstream to increase alertness and energy, is activated. Adrenalin, which is responsible for increasing the heart rate, blood pressure, oxygen into the lungs and dilating pupils, is released. The circulatory system, which pumps oxygen into your heart and lungs and circulates blood through the body, is boosted. Heart rate increases. Breathing is rapid.

Outside: Pupils dilate, body is energetic.

Reaction: To enjoy.

Excited

Meaning: A state of mind and being that elevates you to a high state of joy due to something happening in the past, present or future.

Purpose: To help you enjoy the moment or to help you look forward to future.

Feeling: Happy, enthusiastic.

What happens to the body?

Inside: The brain chemical dopamine, responsible for pleasure and reward, is activated and released. The nervous system, responsible for releasing hormones into the bloodstream, is activated. The hormone adrenalin, which is responsible for increasing heart rate and blood pressure, and getting oxygen into lungs, is released into the bloodstream. The circulatory system, which pumps oxygen into your heart and lungs and circulates blood through the body, is boosted. Heart rate increases. Breathing is rapid.

External: Pupils dilate, sweat beads form, body energizes.

Reaction: To enjoy, to engage, to be motivated.

FULFILLED

Meaning: A state of mind and being that makes you aware that you have achieved something promised, desired or predicted.

Purpose: To help you know you are living a good life and have achieved what you want.

Feeling: Happy, content.

WHAT HAPPENS TO THE MIND AND BODY?

Inside: The brain chemical dopamine, which responsible for pleasure, reward and survival, is activated and released. The brain chemical serotonin, which is responsible for wellbeing and happiness and helps regulate mood and social behaviour, is activated and released. The circulatory system, which pumps oxygen into your heart and lungs and circulates blood through the body, is boosted. The autonomic nervous system, responsible for breathing, heart and digestion, is balanced and regulated. The immune system responsible for defence and protection is regulated.

Outside Eyes brighten, body relaxes.

Reaction: To be complete.

GLAD

Meaning: A state of mind that makes you aware that something good has happened.

Purpose: To make you aware of how you feel about a situation.
Feeling: Glad, pleased, satisfied.

WHAT HAPPENS TO THE BODY?

Inside: The orbitofrontal cortex part of the brain that is strongly connected to senses and processing reward information is activated. The brain chemical dopamine, which is responsible for pleasure and reward, is activated and released. The brain chemical serotonin, which is responsible for regulating mood and social behaviour, is released. The respiratory and circulation system, responsible for breathing and delivering nutrients and oxygen to all cells in the body, is regulated. Heart rate is regulated.

Outside: The mouth forms into a smile or turns upwards.
Reaction: To rejoice.

GRATEFUL

Meaning: A state of mind and being that makes you aware of what you have and what you have been given in your life.
Purpose: To help you be aware of all that you have to help you be aware of the meaning of life; to help you live a life of purpose and passion.
Feeling: Grateful, happy, humble.
Inside: The hypothalamus, which is the part of the brain responsible for regulating sleep, body temperature and feel-good hormones, is activated. The brain chemical dopamine, which is responsible for pleasure and reward, is activated. The brain chemical serotonin, which is responsible for wellbeing and happiness, is activated. The brain chemical oxytocin, which is responsible for social bonding, is triggered. The circulation system, which is responsible for circulating blood nutrients and cells to all of the body, is boosted. The immune system,

responsible for protection and defence, is boosted. Heart rate and breathing is regulated and boosted.

Outside: The body relaxes.

Reaction: To appreciate (know the worth of).

Good

Meaning: A state of mind and being that gives you a sense of wellbeing.

Purpose: To help you see clearly that you are in a good space and place in your life.

Feeling: Happy.

What happens to the body?

Inside: The brain chemical dopamine, which is responsible for pleasure and reward and survival, is activated and released. The brain chemical serotonin, which is responsible for regulating mood and social behaviour, is activated and released. The nervous system that is responsible for outward senses and processing information is balanced and regulated. Heart rate is regulated. Breathing is regulated. Muscles ease and relax.

Outside: Eyes light up, a smile forms.

Reaction: To be (without resistance).

Happy

Meaning: A state of mind and being that makes you aware that you are where you want to be in life.

Purpose: To help you be aware of where you are and where you want to be in your life; to help you be aware of what you want from your life.

Feeling: Content, joy, fulfilled, peaceful, satisfied.

Dictionary

WHAT HAPPENS TO THE BODY?

Inside: The limbic system, which is the portion of the brain responsible for emotions, memories and arousal (stimulation), is activated. The brain chemical dopamine, which is responsible for pleasure, reward and survival, is activated. Endorphins, which are responsible for reducing pain and boosting pleasure, are activated. The brain chemical oxytocin, which is responsible for social bonding and attachments, is activated. The brain chemical serotonin, which is responsible for wellbeing and happiness, is activated and released into the body.T he circulation system, which is responsible for circulating blood nutrients and cells to all of the body, is boosted. The immune system, responsible for protection and defence, is boosted.

Outside: Body is energetic and upbeat.

Reaction: To be (without resistance), to enjoy, to flow.

HOPEFUL

Meaning: A state of mind and being that makes you strongly feel that something will happen and that the situation you are experiencing will move and change.

Purpose: To help you to persevere (to continue in a course of action even in the face of difficulty).

Feeling: Confident.

WHAT HAPPENS TO THE BODY?

Inside: The anterior cingulate cortex, the front part of your brain that is responsible for regulating emotion and decision-making, is activated. The amygdala, which is responsible for your survival instinct and triggers the fight-or-flight response, is activated. Endorphins responsible for reducing pain and boosting pleasure are activated and released into the body.

Heart beat is regulated. Muscles relax.
Outside Body is driven to look forward.
Reaction: To have faith, to trust.

HUMBLE

Meaning: A state of mind and being that places a low significance on all things external that many seem important in life; for example, status, title.

Purpose: To help you to surrender to a life force that is more powerful than yourself.

Feeling: Calm, connected.

WHAT HAPPENS TO THE BODY?

Inside: The cerebellum, which is the part of the brain responsible for posture, balance and coordination, is activated. The brain chemical dopamine, which is responsible for pleasure, reward and survival, is released. The nervous system, responsible for processing information through senses and triggering reactions and actions, is balanced and regulated.

Outside: Body surrenders into whole self.

Reaction: To appreciate, to surrender, to be grateful, to be kind, to be grounded.

INSPIRED

Meaning: A state of mind and being that gives you a surge of energy to feel stimulated with a new and fresh idea or concept.

Purpose: To help you bring something new into existence; to help you expand the limitations of your mind; to help you feel the true feeling of being alive.

Feeling: Enthusiastic, excited.

Dictionary

WHAT HAPPENS TO THE BODY?

Inside: The visual cortex, which is the part of the brain responsible for processing visual information, comes alive. The anterior superior temporal gyrus, which is the part of the brain responsible for processing sounds, is triggered and activated. The brain chemical dopamine, which is responsible for pleasure and reward, is released. The brain chemical serotonin, which is responsible for wellbeing, is activated. Endorphins responsible for reducing pain and boosting pleasure are released into the bloodstream. The circulatory system, which pumps oxygen into your heart and lungs and circulates blood through the body, is boosted. Rapid breathing. Heart rate increases. Blood flow increases.

Outside: Body is energetic and driven to move.

Reaction: To create, to take action.

LOVE

Meaning: An extremely powerful life force that makes you feel connected to someone or something in life that lies beyond yourself.

Purpose: To help you bind, bond, connect, unite.

Feeling: Awe, connected, ecstatic, elated, excited, euphoria, joy, unconditional love.

WHAT HAPPENS TO THE BODY?

Inside: The hypothalamus, the part of the brain responsible for behaviour, hunger, thirst, sleep and sexual response, is activated. The pituitary gland, which is responsible for releasing hormones into the bloodstream, is activated. The brain chemical dopamine, which is responsible for pleasure and reward, is activated. The brain chemical oxytocin, which is responsible for social bonding and attachments, is activated. Phenylethylamine

(PEA), which is an endorphin responsible for energy, alertness and heightened senses and stimulation, is released into the bloodstream. Neutrophils, a family of proteins in your nervous system responsible for signalling neurons and cells to grow and survive, are activated. The endocrine system, which is responsible for stimulating glands, increasing oxygen and glucose, is activated. The blood circulation system, which is responsible for circulating blood nutrients and cells to all of the body, is boosted. Heart rate increases. Rapid breathing. Blood circulation and flow increases.

Outside: Pupils dilate, eyes brighten, skin glows, sweat beads form, body rises.

Reaction: To desire, to attach.

LOVED

Meaning: A state of mind and being that makes you feel you are cared for and looked after; this can be by yourself, by others or by life itself.

Purpose: To help you be aware that you are supported and cared for in life.

Feeling: Happy, secure, safe.

WHAT HAPPENS TO THE BODY?

Inside The brain chemical dopamine, which is responsible for pleasure and reward, is released. The brain chemical serotonin, which is responsible for wellbeing and happiness, is released. The amygdala, which is the part of the brain responsible for activating the fight-or-flight response, decreases. The parasympathetic nervous system, which is part of the body's central nervous system and is responsible for rest and digestion, conserving energy, slowing heart rate down and regulating breathing, is activated. Homeostasis, a

Dictionary

state responsible for body temperature, fluid balance, blood sugar level and stabilizing each cell in your body, is regulated. Muscles relax.

Outside Body is balanced and relaxed.

Reaction: To be (without resistance), to enjoy.

NOSTALGIC

Meaning: A state of mind in which you return to a former time in your life, which helps you remember happy moments.

Purpose: To help you remember the happy moments of your life and help you to see how far you have come in your life.

Feeling: Joy, unconditional love.

WHAT HAPPENS TO THE BODY?

Inside: The hippocampus, the part of the brain responsible for storing life memories and motivation, is activated. The substantia nigra, which is responsible for motor planning and reward planning, is activated. The brain chemical dopamine, which is responsible for pleasure and reward, is released. The brain chemical serotonin, which is responsible for wellbeing and happiness, is released. The circulatory and respiratory systems, which pump oxygen into your heart and lungs and circulate blood through the body, are boosted. Rapid breathing. Heart rate increases. Blood flow increases.

Outside: Body is energized and connects back to life.

Reaction: To reconnect.

OVERJOYED

Meaning: A state of mind and being that allows you to experience great joy and a high level of happiness.

Purpose: To help you be aware that you are deeply enjoying an experience.

Feeling: Delighted, elated, happy, joy.

WHAT HAPPENS TO THE BODY?

Inside: The brain chemical dopamine, which is responsible for pleasure and reward, is activated and released. The brain chemical serotonin, which is responsible for wellbeing and happiness, is released. Endorphins, which are responsible for reducing pain and increasing pleasure, are released into the bloodstream. The circulation system, which is responsible for circulating blood nutrients and cells to all of the body, is boosted. The immune system, responsible for protection and defence, is boosted. Heart rate increases. Rapid breathing. Blood flows increases.

Outside: Pupils dilate, skin is flushed, mouth forms into a smile.

Reaction: To take action, to jump for joy.

PASSIONATE

Meaning: A state of mind and being that gives you a strong driving force toward something or someone.

Purpose: To help you understand what you want and help you to act upon it.

Feeling: Enthusiastic, eager, excited.

WHAT HAPPENS TO THE BODY?

Inside: The ventral striatum, which is part of the limbic system and is responsible for decision making and reward-related behaviour is activated. (The limbic system is the portion of the brain that deals with emotions, memories and arousal.) The amygdala, which is the part of the brain responsible for emotions and survival, is activated. The hippocampus, the part of the brain responsible for motivation, emotion and learning, is activated. The circulatory system, which is responsible for circulating blood to the heart and lungs and through the entire body and is also responsible for delivering nutrients and oxygen to all cells in the body, is boosted. Heart rate increases. Breathing is rapid.

Outside: Pupils dilate, eyes widen, skin flushes, body is energetic.

Reaction: To desire, to be motivated, to show interest.

PATIENT

Meaning: A mental state of mind and being in which you accept any situation without complaint or annoyance, no matter how difficult, painful, disturbing or turbulent it may be for you.

Purpose: To help you to move through uncomfortable situations with ease; to help you stop resisting or pushing forward too quickly and connect with the power of life.

Feeling: Calm.

WHAT HAPPENS TO THE BODY?

Inside: The task positive network – the region of the brain responsible for activation, increase in attention and demanding tasks – is activated. The brain chemical serotonin, which is responsible for regulating your mood and social bonding, is activated and released into the body. Breathing is regulated.

Outside: Body is in balance, body is steady.

Reaction: To surrender (stop resisting).

PEACEFUL

Meaning: A state of mind and being where you are free from any forms of stress, trouble or disturbances influenced by internal and external forces.

Purpose: To help you to come back in alignment with your natural state; to help you connect with your true nature.

Feeling: Calm, content, carefree, comfortable, happy, serene, safe.

WHAT HAPPENS TO THE BODY?

Inside: The insular cortex, which is the part of the brain involved perception, motor control, self-awareness and regulating the body's homeostasis, is activated. The brain chemical gamma aminobutyric acid gaba, which is responsible for the calming activity and reducing nervous activity, is activated and released into the body. The nervous system that is responsible for processing information through senses and triggering reactions is balanced and regulated. The parasympathetic nervous system, which is responsible for rest and digestion and conserving energy, is activated. Heart rate is regulated. Breathing is regulated. Blood flow increases. Muscles ease and relax

Outside: Body is relaxed, body is steady.

Reaction: To be (without resistance), to flow, to surrender.

PLAYFUL

Meaning: A state of mind and being where you are feeling pure pleasure in the moment of your experience.

Purpose: To help you connect; to help you create.

Feeling: Happy, energetic, enthusiastic, joy.

WHAT HAPPENS TO THE BODY?

Inside: The frontal lobe, which is the part of your brain responsible for expression, problem-solving, memory, language, judgement and behaviours, is activated. The striatum, which is the front brain responsible for motor skills and voluntary movement, is activated. The thalamic nuclei, which is the part of the brain responsible for sensory and motor signals, is triggered. The brain chemical dopamine, which is responsible for pleasure and reward, is released into the body. Endorphins, which are responsible for reducing pain and boosting pleasure, are released into the bloodstream. The circulation system, which is responsible for circulating blood nutrients and cells to all of the body, is boosted. The immune system, which is responsible for protection and defence, is boosted. Heart rate increases. Rapid breathing. Blood flow increases.

Outside: Body is energetic, body moves with ease.

Reaction: To enjoy, to be free.

PLEASED

Meaning: A feeling of pleasure, especially with an event or a situation.

Purpose: To help you have a pleasurable experience.

Feeling: Satisfied, glad, content.

WHAT HAPPENS TO THE BODY?

Inside: The orbitofrontal cortex part of the brain that is strongly connected to external senses and processing reward information is activated. The brain chemical dopamine, which is responsible for pleasure and reward, is activated and released. The brain chemical messenger serotonin, which is responsible for regulating mood and social behaviour, is activated and released. The respiratory and circulation systems, responsible for regulating breathing and delivering nutrients and oxygen to all cells in the body, are activated.

Outside: Body relaxes.

Reaction: To approve (accept as satisfactory).

POWERFUL

Meaning: A mental state of mind and being that allows you to be capable of producing great effects and results.

Purpose: To help you to tap into your inner self; to help you to apply and gather all of your inner strengths and forces so you can be fully capable of seeing a situation through.

Feeling: Confident, courageous, connected, decisive, dedicated, enthusiastic, focused, inspired, passionate.

WHAT HAPPENS TO THE BODY?

Inside: The left frontal cortex, which is the part of the brain responsible for controlling language and movement, is activated. The prefrontal cortex, which is the part of the brain responsible for your personality, development, expression, planning, action, decision-making, execution, organizing and monitoring results, is activated. The ventral striatum, which is the part of the brain responsible for decision-making and reward-related behaviour, is activated. The brain chemical dopamine, which is responsible for pleasure and reward, is activated. The brain chemical oxytocin, which is responsible for social bonding, is activated. Noradrenaline, the hormone responsible for mobilizing the brain and body for action, is activated. The circulatory system, which is responsible for circulating blood through the body and regulating the heart and oxygen, is boosted. Heart rate increases. Rapid breathing. Blood flow increases.

Outside: The body rises high and stands strong, speech is strong and clear.

Reaction: To influence (to shape or to have an effect on behaviours, situations, developments, and outcomes).

RELAXED

Meaning: A state of being that relieves you from any type of tension, stress or anxiety.

Purpose: To help you to let go.

Feeling: Calm, comfortable, happy, safe, secure.

WHAT HAPPENS TO THE BODY?

Inside: The brain activates into a default mode network, which means large areas of the brain go on standby. The default brain network is responsible for wakeful rest. The parasympathetic nervous system – which is part of the central nervous system and is responsible for rest and digestion by conserving energy, slowing heart rate, breathing and increased digestion – is activated and stimulated. The brain chemical gamma-aminobutyric acid gaba, which is responsible for calming activity and reducing nervous activity, is activated and released into the body. The brain chemical oxytocin, which is responsible for boosting the immune system and reducing stress hormones, is activated and released into the body and bloodstream.

Outside: Body is at ease.

Reaction: To be (without resistance), to enjoy, to surrender.

RELIEVED

Meaning: A state of mind and being that allows you to release from any form of tension, pain or distress.

Purpose: To help you release stress and return back to your natural state of being.

Feeling: Happy, joy.

WHAT HAPPENS TO THE BODY?

Inside: The parasympathetic nervous system, which is part of the central nervous system and helps the body rest by conserving energy and slowing down the heart rate, is activated. The respiratory system, which is responsible for your breathing, is reset as the lungs increase for the intake of oxygen.

Outside: Body relaxes and sighs.
Reaction: To relax.

RESTFUL

Meaning: A state of mind and being where you cease work or movement in order to relax, sleep, recharge or recover strength.
Purpose: To help you to restore to a natural state and help you to regain strength.
Feeling: Relaxed, calm, tranquil, peaceful.
WHAT HAPPENS TO THE BODY?
Inside: The parasympathetic nervous system, which is responsible for rest, conserving energy, slowing heart rate, relaxing muscles and increasing digestion, is activated. Cortisol levels and stress hormones decrease. The homeostasis state, which helps body temperature, fluid balance and blood sugar level stabilize and balances each cell in the body, is regulated. Breath is regulated. Heart rate and digestion is regulated. Muscles ease and relax.
Outside: Body is boosted.
Reaction: To be (without resistance).

SAFE

Meaning: A state of mind and being that makes you feel secure and free from any threat, hurt, harm, injury, danger or risk.
Purpose: To help you feel secure and live a life without fear.
Feeling: Happy, comfortable, connected, peaceful, joy.
WHAT HAPPENS TO THE BODY?
Inside: The brain chemical serotonin, which is responsible for wellbeing and happiness, is released. The brain chemical dopamine, which is responsible for pleasure and reward, is activated and

released. The nervous system, responsible for fight and flight, goes on standby and sets your body in a homeostasis state. The parasympathetic nervous system, which is part of the central nervous system and is responsible for the body's ability to rest, is activated. Heart rate is regulated. Energy is conserved. The respiratory and circulation systems, responsible for breathing and delivering nutrients and oxygen to all cells in the body, are regulated.

Outside: Body is balanced and stable.

Reaction: To be (without resistance), to trust.

SATISFIED

Meaning: A state of mind and being that makes you feel that an expectation, a need, a desire or a demand has been met.

Purpose: To help you experience the simple pleasures that life has to offer you.

Feeling: Content, fulfilled, glad, happy, pleased, joy.

WHAT HAPPENS TO THE BODY?

Inside: The brain chemical dopamine, which is responsible for pleasure and reward, is activated and released. The brain chemical oxytocin, which is responsible for social bonding, is activated. The brain chemical serotonin, which is responsible for happiness and wellbeing, is activated. The circulatory system, which is responsible for circulating blood to the heart and lungs and delivering nutrients to all cells in the body, is regulated.

Outside: Body is relaxed.

Reaction: To enjoy.

SECURE

Meaning: A state of mind and being that makes you feel that you are positioned firmly and correctly and, therefore, not likely to move, fall or break.

Purpose: To help you to feel safe.

Feeling: Comfortable, happy, relaxed, safe.

WHAT HAPPENS TO THE BODY?

Inside: The parasympathetic nervous system, which is part of the central nervous system and helps rest by conserving energy and slowing down heart rate, is activated. The brain chemical serotonin, which is responsible for wellbeing and happiness, is released. The brain chemical dopamine, which is responsible for social bonding, is activated and released. The respiratory and circulation systems, responsible for breathing and delivering nutrients and oxygen to all cells in the body, are regulated.

Outside: Body is relaxed and moves easily and freely.

Reaction: To trust.

SURPRISED

Meaning: A mental state of mind and being that makes you aware that something unexpected has happened.

Purpose: To help you shift out of your current state; to help you be aware that something is happening that you did not expect.

Feeling: Astonished, startled.

WHAT HAPPENS TO THE BODY?

Inside: The hippocampus, which is the part of the brain responsible for emotion, learning and memory, is stimulated and activated. The neural pathway, which is a collection of nerves that are connected and travel through the body, is instantly activated. The mesolimbic pathway, which is the pathway in the brain that releases the brain chemical dopamine, responds instantly. The brain chemical dopamine, which is responsible for stimulating arousal and causing excitement, is activated. The circulation system, which is responsible for circulating blood, nutrients and cells to all of the body, is boosted. The

Dictionary

immune system, which is responsible for protection and defence, is boosted. Heart rate increases. Rapid breathing. Blood flow increases.

Outside: Eyes widen, eyebrows raise, jaw drops.

Reaction: To change view, to change perspective.

TRANQUIL

Meaning: A state of mind in which you are free of any disturbance.

Purpose: To help you to truly be and feel free in that moment of your life.

Feeling: Bliss, calm, peaceful.

WHAT HAPPENS TO THE BODY?

Inside: The respiratory control centre, which is part of the brain responsible for generating and maintaining the rhythm of respiration and adjusting the balance in your cells, is activated. The parasympathetic nervous system, which is part of the central nervous system and helps the body to rest by conserving energy and slowing down heart rate, is activated. Muscle tensions ease.

Outside: Body is loose and moves freely.

Reaction: To relax, to surrender (stop resisting).

THRILLED

Meaning: A state of mind and being that moves you into a sudden sensation of intense excitement, joy and pleasure.

Purpose: To help you experience a rush of joy; to help you feel alive.

Feeling: Excited, overjoyed.

WHAT HAPPENS TO THE BODY?

Inside: The brain chemical dopamine, which is responsible for pleasure and reward, is activated and released. The nervous system, which is responsible for processing external sensory information and triggering reactions, is activated. Adrenalin, which is responsible for increasing the heart rate, raising blood pressure, increasing oxygen into the lungs and increasing blood sugar levels, is activated. The circulatory system, which is responsible for circulating blood to the heart and lungs, is boosted. Heart rate increases. Body temperature increases. Breathing increases. Blood flows out.

Outside: Body trembles and tingles.

Reaction: Move up and down.

WONDER

Meaning: A state of mind that makes you feel an intense emotional reaction to an unexpected phenomenon.

Purpose: To help you perceive and experience something extraordinary and beautiful.

Feeling: Amazed, awe, astonished.

WHAT HAPPENS TO THE BODY?

Inside: The hippocampus, which is the part of the brain responsible for emotion, learning and memory, is stimulated and activated. The brain chemical dopamine, which is responsible for pleasure and reward, is released. The brain chemical serotonin, which is responsible for wellbeing, is released. Endorphins, which are responsible for reducing pain and boosting pleasure, is triggered and then released into the bloodstream. The circulatory system, which is responsible for pumping oxygen into your heart and lungs and circulating blood through the body, is boosted. Heart rate increases. Breathing increases.

Outside: Pupils dilate, eyes widen, body rises.

Reaction: To admire.

Dictionary

Positive reactions and responses

When you feel naturally good inside your mind and body, you may experience some of the following reactions and responses. If you are unaware of how you feel, and cannot pinpoint it or find a name, be aware of and see your reaction; this can help you to understand how you really feel on the inside, and what is happening to you on the outside.

REACTION	RESPONSE
Action	act upon
Admire	regard with respect or warm approval
Accept	receive
Affinity	a natural liking or understanding of someone or something
Attach	be a part of
Appreciate	know the worth
Balanced	in good proportion – mind, body and spirit
Be	allow yourself to exist (without resistance)
Believe	accept as true
Bind	tie together
Bond	a strong force of attraction
Brave	ready to face and endure danger or pain
Complete	all of
Connect	feel an affinity to life, to people, to places, to the world
Create	act upon
Creative	use your imagination
Desire	want
Embrace	open up and bring closer
Enjoy	take pleasure in
Eustress	collection of nerves collated to help push your mind and body forward
Explore	want to know more
Faith	have complete trust confidence in something

REACTION	RESPONSE
Flow	move along in a steady, continuous stream
Free	flow freely
Gesture	move to express
Engage	have an interest or enthusiasm
Give	offer something
Influence	have power
Motivated	desire to have an effect on behaviours, situations, developments, and outcomes
Persevere	continue in a course of action even in the face of difficulty
Plan	make arrangements
Play	engage in activity for pleasure, enjoyment
Prepare	start to get ready
Proud	feeling of deep pleasure and satisfaction
Relax	loosen up
Significance	give attention to
Steady	firmly fixed
Surrender	stop resisting
Trust	believe in
Unite	come together

If you feel good in your mind and body, it is natural for you to:

- admire
- accept
- connect
- enjoy
- trust
- feel safe
- surrender
- relax
- unite

A final note on positive

There will be times in your life when your mind and body will move away from positive. If this happens, this means your mind and body are being pushed through spaces and places, phases, stages, events, environments and circumstances that are testing, challenging or disconnecting you in some way. This can prevent you from feeling good or experiencing any positive states. If this happens, and you lose your way into a deep, negative state and cannot find your way back to positive, always remember there are two natural states that lie at the root of positive states. These two states are:

- joy
- unconditional love

As mentioned at the start of the chapter, they are always with you, waiting to reveal themselves to you. They lie waiting for you beneath all your life experiences. When you are ready to feel good again, these two positive emotions will naturally unveil themselves to you and your mind, and your body will feel connected to life and the joy of life and the love of life again.

Note: If it has been a long time since you have felt positive, do what you can to place your mind and body in neutral. This will help you to connect to your whole self, find balance, and see clearly.

THE BLANK CANVAS: POSITIVE

Each time you find yourself visiting the Positive dictionary because you have experienced one of the emotions or feelings above, and you have sat with the emotion or feeling, then take a moment to place the name of the feeling (or even just a tick) in the circle to remind yourself of that positive feeling.

Positive:

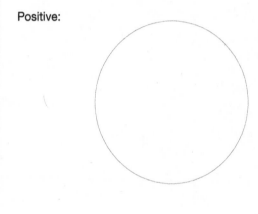

5

DICTIONARY OF FEELINGS – NEUTRAL

Neutral states of mind and being are here to help you to:

- be still
- be steady
- gain clarity
- observe life
- stay balanced
- stay calm
- stay neutral
- be connected to life and the nature of life

Being neutral

When your mind and body enter into a neutral state, this means you are experiencing neutral events, circumstances, situations and outcomes. These will NOT stir energy, emotion or feeling.

When your mind and body shifts to a neutral state and channels this energy to your body, you will feel calm, balanced. Your life lens will be clear.

A neutral state of mind and being will help you to stay balanced, especially during times of disruption, movement and change. A neutral state of mind and being will help you to find your way back to your whole self again when you lose your way.

EQUANIMITY
Meaning: A state of mind and being that is undisturbed by experience or emotion.
Purpose: To keep your mind and body balanced, especially during uncomfortable and difficult situations.
Feeling: Calm.
WHAT HAPPENS TO THE BODY?
Inside: The prefrontal cortex, which is the part of the brain responsible for monitoring emotions, is activated. The parasympathetic nervous system, which is responsible for the body's rest and digestion, is activated. The sympathetic nervous system, which is responsible for stimulating the body's fight-or-flight response, goes on standby. The brain chemical serotonin, which is responsible for happiness and wellbeing, is activated. The brain chemical GABA, which is responsible for regulating excited nerves, is activated. The basal ganglia, which is responsible for the control of voluntary motor movements, procedural learning, habit learning, eye movements and cognition, eases. Cingulate gyrus, which is responsible for processing emotions and behaviour regulation, stabilizes. Energy is conserved. Heart rate lowers. Muscles relax. Breathing is regulated.
Outside: Body is balanced and steady.
Reaction: To compose, to have faith, to observe, to trust.

EQUILIBRIUM
Meaning: A mental state that will place all your emotions into balance; a state of balance between two opposing forces.

Purpose: To keep you steady; to be aware of any emotion or feeling that comes up within your physical body so you do not deny, suppress or suffocate them.

Feeling: Calm.

WHAT HAPPENS TO THE BODY?

Inside: The cerebellum, the part of the brain which controls balance, coordination and fine muscle control and posture, is activated. The brain chemical GABA, which is responsible for regulating excited nerves, is activated. The parasympathetic nervous system, which is responsible for the body's rest and digestion, is activated. The sympathetic nervous system, which is responsible for stimulating the body's fight-or-flight response, goes on standby. Heart rate regulates. Breathing regulates.

Outside: Body is in balance.

Reaction: To observe, to be mindful.

NEUTRAL

Meaning: A state of mind and being that places you in neutral space.

Purpose: To help you to connect and flow with the energy that is your life.

Feeling: Calm, relaxed.

WHAT HAPPENS TO THE BODY?

Inside: The default network, which is the part of the brain responsible for wakeful rest, is activated. The parasympathetic nervous system, which is responsible for the body's rest and digestion, is activated. The sympathetic nervous system, which is responsible for stimulating the body's fight-or-flight response, goes on standby. The brain chemical GABA, which is responsible for regulating excited nerves, is activated.

Outside: Body is in balance.

Reaction: To be present, to observe.

Neutral reactions and responses

When you feel naturally balanced in your mind and body – in a neutral state – you may experience some of the following reactions and responses.

REACTION	RESPONSE
Compose	settle
Faith	complete trust or confidence in something
Observe	watch carefully
Trust	believe something is safe and reliable
Mindful	conscious and aware
Present	existing or occurring now

A final note on neutral

If you have lost your way deep in positive or negative states, or if your mind is being disturbed or disrupted or clouded by emotions, and you cannot think or see clearly or understand what you are feeling, a neutral state of mind and being can help you to see clearly and gain perspective.

There are ways to help move your mind and body back into a homeostasis and balanced state again, which are explored in an earlier chapter.

THE BLANK CANVAS: NEUTRAL

Each time you find yourself visiting the Neutral dictionary because you have experienced one of the emotions or feelings above, and you have sat with the emotion or feeling, take a moment to place the name of the feeling (or even just a tick) in the circle to remind yourself of that feeling.

Neutral:

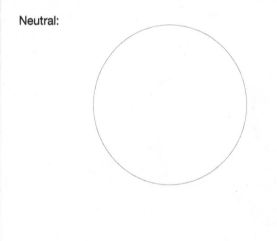

6

DICTIONARY OF FEELINGS – NEGATIVE

Negative states are here to help:

- protect your mind and body from threatening or dangerous situations
- protect your mind and body from situations that threaten your wellbeing
- push your mind and body out of a comfortable state so you can grow
- push you to develop, grow and evolve to the next stage of your life

Being negative

When your mind and body enter into a negative state, this means you are experiencing negative events, circumstances, situations and outcomes. These will stir negative energy, emotions or feelings.

This energy will channel its way into the body and start to feel like a feeling of alert, alarm, discomfort and/or pain.

When your mind and body shifts to a negative state, your mind will shift from a place of comfort to a place of discomfort. Your life lens will be cloudy and pessimistic.

Negative feelings can range from mild to very strong, and your vibration or mood will be low. If It is a first-time experience, it can feel mild; if this is a recurring or repeated experience, and if you are not aware of the emotion or feeling inside you and it keeps resurfacing over time, it will feel stronger and louder inside you, and this strength will feel more painful.

WORK WITH

It is vital for your wellbeing that you allow negative states to arise naturally. They have arisen in your mind for a reason, so if you observe and are aware what is rising in you, you can work _with_ what is happening to you.

WORK AGAINST

Negative states are uncomfortable and painful, and do not feel good in mind and body. You may feel an instant urge to resist, dismiss, reject, suppress, block, bury, hide, deny or push away the negative emotion and feelings altogether. You may do so to avoid feeling discomfort or internal pain, and want to move away from this state as quickly as possible. Do not do this. If you refuse to see and work with the negative state, it will not move away: it will reside inside you and resurface at another time in your life.

A negative emotion or feeling can cause a negative reaction that you may try to act against – this can cause a negative chain reaction, which can have extremely negative consequences. This is why it is vital you take time out to understand how you feel If you regularly experience negative states of mind and being. If you are continuously reacting from a negative space and experiencing internal reactions from external situations, please seek professional help or speak to a friend.

The root

There are two natural states that lie at the root of negative states:

- fear
- sadness

They are always with you, waiting to reveal themselves to you. These states lie waiting for you beneath all your life experiences.

FEAR

Meaning: A powerful state of mind and being that tells your mind and body that there is a threat that can be harmful or dangerous.

Purpose: To help you be aware you are not safe; to help you stay alert so you can protect yourself from harm and danger; to help steer you away from harmful or dangerous situations.

Feeling: Afraid.

WHAT HAPPENS TO THE BODY?

Inside: The amygdala, the part of the brain responsible for receiving incoming messages, receives a message of threat and danger and sends a message to the hypothalamus, which immediately triggers the fight-or-flight response. The front lobe, which is the part of the brain responsible for personality, problem-solving and behaviour, is shut down. The pituitary gland, which releases stress hormones, is activated. The sympathetic nervous system, which prepares the body for fight and flight, is activated. The stress hormone cortisol, which increases energy in the bloodstream, is released. Adrenalin, which distributes blood to muscles, is released. Noradrenaline, responsible for alertness and mobilizing brain and body for action, is released. The immune, digestive and reproductive systems are suppressed or shut down. Heart rate speeds up. Rapid breathing. Blood pressure rises. Blood vessels constrict. Muscles tighten and tense. Peripheral vision is lost, causing tunnel vision. Hearing decreases.

Outside: Pupils dilate, sweat beads form, body is on high alert – ready for action.

Reaction: Your body will be ready to fight or flight (instantly move away). Continuous activation of the fight-or-flight response will disrupt your sympathetic and parasympathetic nervous systems, which work together to help keep your body balanced. You will be in misalignment and disharmony, and this can lead you on to a path of destruction and self-destruction.

Power: To protect and disconnect.

Vibration: Low.

SADNESS

Meaning: A state of mind and being that is influenced and impacted by an awareness of change, loss, pain and suffering.

Purpose: To help you be aware of life and the changes that come with life.

Feeling: Sad.

WHAT HAPPENS TO THE BODY?

Inside: The cerebrum – the largest part of the brain and responsible for thinking and feeling, as well as emotion and awareness – registers that something bad is happening or changing. The hippocampus, responsible for storing memory, is activated. The amygdala, responsible for emotions and behaviour, is activated. The hypothalamus, which is connected to your autonomic nervous system and regulates your breathing, heartbeat and digestion, is triggered. The parasympathetic nervous system, which slows heart rate and increases gland activity, is activated. The hormone acetylcholine, responsible for dilating blood vessels and increasing bodily secretion, is released.

The feel-good chemicals dopamine and serotonin decrease. The lachrymal gland, which produces tears, is triggered. Global sensation, which causes a lump in the throat, is activated. Heart rate decreases. Breath decreases. Muscles contract.

Outside: Tears form in the eyes, lump forms in throat, nose waters, posture slumps, body movement slows down.

Reaction: To cry.

Power: You will be be aware and release. When you reveal or release your sadness, something will shift inside of you; when you feel that release, that moment of setting yourself free, you move one step closer to positive again and unconditional love.

Vibration: Low.

The layers

*Warning:
If any of these emotions are severe and keep repeating themselves, please seek professional help.

ANGRY

Meaning: A state of mind and being that makes you feel you are treated in an unfair, cruel and unacceptable way.

Purpose: To give you strength and help you to find a way to make a change.

Feeling: Annoyed, irritated, uncomfortable. (Anger can layer over hurt and hate.)

WHAT HAPPENS TO THE BODY?

Inside: The amygdala, the part of the brain responsible for receiving messages from senses, receives a message of a threat. The front lobe of the brain, responsible for personality, problem-solving and behaviour, is shut down. The hypothalamus,

Dictionary

which is connected to your autonomic nervous system and unconsciously regulates your breathing, heartbeat and digestion, is triggered. The sympathetic nervous system, which stimulates the body's fight-or-flight response, is activated. The stress hormone cortisol, responsible for mood, motivation, emotions and alerting or shutting down bodily functions such as the digestive, immune, and reproductive systems or growth processes, is released. Adrenalin, which distributes blood to muscles in readiness for action, is released. The hormone noradrenaline, which mobilizes the brain and body for action, is released. Heart rate increases. Rapid breathing. Blood pressure increases. Muscles contract. Blood vessels constrict.

Outside: Pupils dilate, senses heighten, body is energized.

Reaction: You will want to act or react. Anger is a powerful force; if not handled with care, and if you lash out to release this force without thinking, it can cause damage and destruction, sometimes beyond repair.

Root cause: Fear, sadness.

ANGUISH

Meaning: A state of mind and being where you feel a deep mental or emotional pain through some form of suffering (pain, distress or hardship).

Purpose: To help you to understand free will (choosing between different causes of action).

Feeling: Anxiety, hurt, despair, distress, unhappy, grief, sorrow.

WHAT HAPPENS TO THE BODY?

Inside: The cerebral cortex, the part of the brain responsible for processing information and perceiving life events, is activated. The somatosensory cortex, the part of the brain that receives and processes sensory information from the entire body, is activated. The anterior insula, the part of the brain responsible for sensory signals and feeling sensations in the body, is activated. The anterior cingulate cortex, the part of the brain responsible for regulating emotions and processing pain, is activated. The sympathetic nervous system, which is responsible for the fight-or-flight response, is activated. The stress hormone cortisol, responsible for mood, motivation, emotions and alerting or shutting down bodily functions such as the digestive, immune and reproductive systems, is released into the bloodstream. Heart rate increases. Rapid breathing. Blood pressure increases. Muscles contract. Blood vessels constrict.

Outside: Face and body crumple.

Reaction: To be devastated.

Root Cause: Fear, sadness.

ANTICIPATION (NB: THIS CAN ALSO BE A POSITIVE MENTAL STATE)

Meaning: A mental state of mind and being that is waiting, predicting or expecting an outcome of an event or situation that will not feel good.

Purpose: To help you be aware that you are scared of an outcome.

Feeling: Anxious, nervous.

WHAT HAPPENS TO THE BODY?

Inside: The amygdala – the part of the brain responsible for receiving incoming messages from senses – receives a message of a threat. The anterior cingulate cortex – the part of the brain responsible for processing emotions, attention and decision-making – and the sympathetic nervous system, which stimulates the body's fight-or-flight response, are activated. The hormone adrenalin, which keeps the body energized and alert, is activated. The stress hormone cortisol, which helps the body respond to stress, is activated. Rapid breathing. Heart rate increases. Blood vessels constrict. Muscles contract. Blood flow decreases.

Outside: Body is tense.

Reaction: To be restless.

Root Cause: Fear.

ANIMOSITY

Meaning: A state of mind and being where you experience a strong feeling of dislike towards something or someone.

Purpose: To help you be aware that you do not like something.

Feeling: Hate.

WHAT HAPPENS TO THE BODY?

Inside: The amygdala, which is the part of the brain responsible for receiving incoming messages, receives a message of threat. The autonomic nervous system, which triggers fight or flight and releases the stress hormones cortisol and adrenalin into the bloodstream, is triggered. Heart rate speeds up. Rapid breathing. Blood pressure rises. Blood vessels constrict. Muscles tighten and tense.

Outside: Body is tense and uptight.

Reaction: To resist.

Root Cause: Fear.

ANNOYED

Meaning: An unpleasant mental state of mind caused by a disturbance from something or someone.

Purpose: To help you be aware that something is getting in your way of getting what you want or in the way of where you want to be.

Feeling: Frustration, irritated, angry.

WHAT HAPPENS TO THE BODY?

Inside: The cerebrum left hemisphere of the brain, which is responsible for logical and performance tasks, sends a message to the body that it is being disturbed. The amygdala, which is the emotional centre of the brain, is activated and sends a message to the hypothalamus. The hypothalamus actions the release of hormones, and the fight-or-flight response is activated. The hormone cortisol, which responds to stress, is activated. The sympathetic nervous system, responsible for fight or flight, is activated. The heart rate increases. The blood flow increases. Muscles tense up.

Outside: Body is tense and uptight.

Reaction: To be agitated, to be troubled.

Root Cause: Fear.

APPREHENSIVE

Meaning: A state of mind and being that makes you feel that something bad or unpleasant may happen in the future.

Purpose: To help you to be aware that you are not looking forward to something and are scared to experience it.

Feeling: Worried, anxious, disturbed.

WHAT HAPPENS TO THE BODY?

Inside: The anterior cingulate cortex, which is the part of the brain responsible for emotion, attention and decision-making, is activated and sends a message to the body that a potentially threatening situation may take place. Adrenalin, which keeps the body energized and alert, is activated and released into the bloodstream. The steroid hormone cortisol, which helps the body respond to stress, is activated and released into the bloodstream. The sympathetic nervous system, which stimulates the body's fight-or-flight response, is activated. Heart beat is rapid. Muscles tighten and contract.

Outside: The body is restless.

Reaction: To be restless.

Root Cause: Fear.

ANXIOUS

Meaning: A state of mind and being that places you in an unpleasant state of inner turmoil.

Purpose: To help your mind and body be on high alert for threat or danger.

Feeling: Anticipation, nervous, uncomfortable, worried, uneasy.

WHAT HAPPENS TO THE BODY?

Inside: The amygdala, which is the part of the brain responsible for responding to fear, becomes overactive. The hypothalamus activates the sympathetic nervous system by sending signals through the autonomic nerves to the adrenal glands. The sympathetic nervous system, which prepares the body for fight and flight, is activated. The pituitary gland, which releases stress hormones, is activated. Cortisol, which increases energy, is released in the bloodstream. Adrenalin, which distributes blood to muscles, is released. Noradrenaline, which is responsible for alertness and mobilizing brain and body for action, is released. The immune, digestive and reproductive systems are suppressed or shut down. Heart rate speeds up. Rapid breathing. Blood pressure rises. Blood vessels constrict. Muscles tighten and tense. Peripheral vision is lost, causing tunnel vision. Hearing decreases.

Outside: Dizziness, shortness of breath, sweating, trembling, chest tightness.

Reaction: To be hyperactive, to be on high alert, to be restless.

Root Cause: Fear.

BITTER

Meaning: A state of being where you are aware you had a bad experience and you cannot forget what happened – the feeling lingers and resides inside of you.

Purpose: To help you be aware that you are stuck in the experience and cannot move forward.

Feeling: Angry, hurt, hatred, pain, powerless, resentment, sadness.

WHAT HAPPENS TO THE BODY?

Inside: The hippocampus, which is the part of the brain responsible for repeating life memories, is activated. The amygdala, which processes emotions, is over-activated. The thalamus, which triggers emotions connected to past events, is activated. The somatosensory cortex, which is a part of the brain that receives and processes sensory information from the entire body, is activated. Homeostatic regulation, which controls the balance of cells in your body, gets disrupted. The endocrine system, which releases hormones into the bloodstream and works in balance with the immune system and nervous system, is unregulated. The cardiovascular system, which pumps blood to the heart and brain, is irregular. The respiratory system, which helps you breathe, is irregular. Heart rate and breath are irregular. Muscles tighten and constrict. Blood flow is restricted.

Outside: Body is tense.

Reaction: To belittle, to resent, to spite, to be vindictive.

Root Cause: Fear, sadness.

BORED

Meaning: A state of mind and being that makes you feel restless because you do not have anything interesting to do.

Purpose: To help you to stop thinking; to help you become

Dictionary

creative; to help you be inspired – being bored, if worked with, can help you to explore your whole self and others in ways you would not do if you were busy.

Feeling: Unhappy.

WHAT HAPPENS TO THE BODY?

Inside: The cerebrum – which is the largest part of the brain and responsible for thinking and feeling, as well as emotion and awareness – registers that the mind and body have nothing to do. The amygdala, which is the part of the brain responsible for emotions and behaviour, is activated. The hypothalamus part of your brain, which is connected to your autonomic nervous system and regulates your breathing, heartbeat and digestion, is triggered. The sympathetic nervous system, which prepares the body for fight and flight, is activated. The stress hormone cortisol, which increases energy, is released into the bloodstream. Adrenalin, which distributes blood to muscles, is released. Rapid breathing. Blood pressure rises. Blood vessels constrict. Muscles tighten and tense.

Outside: Body is restless.

Reaction: To be restless.

Root Cause: Fear.

CONFLICTED

Meaning: A mental state of mind and being where you do not know what to think or feel because of inconsistent emotions, ideas, opinions, thoughts and beliefs.

Purpose: To help you to be aware that you do not know the way and are uncertain

Feeling: Confused.

What happens to the body?

Inside: The prefrontal cortex – which is the part of the brain that detects sense of self and value systems, and is responsible for our self-control – fires messages back and forth to the amygdala. The amygdala, which is the emotional centre of the brain, receives the continuous messages as a potential threat and sends a message to the hypothalamus. The hypothalamus, which releases hormones and actions the flight-or-fight response, sends a message to the body to prepare for a threat. The steroid hormone cortisol, which deals with stress and shutting down other bodily functions (such as the immune system, the reproductive system and growth), is activated and released into the bloodstream. Breathing is restricted. Blood flow is reduced. Muscles tighten.

Outside: Body is restless, tense, uptight.

Reaction: To be restless.

Root Cause: Fear.

Confused

Meaning: A state of mind and being where you are unable to think clearly or understand what is happening to you.

Purpose: To help you be aware that you do not know where you are or what you are doing.

Feeling: Conflicted, uneasy, uncomfortable.

What happens to the body?

Inside: The prefrontal cortex, which is the part of the brain responsible for attention and focus, fires messages back and forth to the amygdala. The amygdala sends continuous messages of a potential threat to the hypothalamus. The hypothalamus, which is the part of the brain responsible for releasing hormones and actioning the flight-or-fight response, sends a message to the body to prepare for a threat. The autonomic nervous system, which regulates your heart, breathing, digestion, and pupil responses, activates your sympathetic nervous system. The sympathetic nervous system triggers the fight-or-flight response. The stress hormones cortisol and adrenalin are released into the bloodstream. Blood vessels constrict. Muscles tense. Heartbeat and breathing are irregular. Sweat glands are overactive.

Outside: Body is restless, head is unclear and can ache.

Reaction: To be uncertain.

Root Cause: Fear, sadness.

DEFEATED

Meaning: A state of mind or being where you feel you have been beaten, worn down or demoralized.

Purpose: To help you to surrender (stop resisting).

Feeling: Powerless.

WHAT HAPPENS TO THE BODY?

Inside: The amygdala, which is the part of the brain responsible for emotions and behaviour, is activated. The hypothalamus, which is the part of your brain connected to your autonomic nervous system and regulates your breathing, heartbeat and digestion is triggered. The parasympathetic nervous system, which is responsible for slowing heart rate and increasing gland activity, is activated. Heart rate decreases. Breath decreases. Muscles contract.

Outside: Body lowers, posture slumps.

Reaction: To give up.

Root Cause: Sadness.

DEPRESSED

Meaning: A state of mind and being that makes you feel so low that you are unable to deal with a situation or with life itself.

Purpose: To help you be aware that you have lost connection with yourself, your spirit and your life.

Feeling: Anguish, confused, conflicted, defeated, distressed, hopeless, unhappy.

WHAT HAPPENS TO THE BODY?

Inside: The amygdala, which is the part of the brain responsible for perception and assessment of the environment, sends a message to the thalamus that it is not feeling good. The thalamus, which is responsible for receiving sensory information, signals the cerebral cortex. The cerebral cortex, which is responsible for thinking, perceiving, producing and understanding language, receives the information that the brain is receiving a negative state. The hippocampus, which is the part of the brain responsible for storing memories, triggers past memories so your body can prepare. The feel-good brain chemicals serotonin and dopamine, responsible for wellbeing, pleasure and reward, decrease. The brain chemical norepinephrine, which mobilizes the brain and body for action, decreases. There will be a lack of energy and disturbance of appetite and sleep. The digestive, immune and reproductive systems are irregular. Heartbeat is irregular. Breathing decreases. Blood pressure increases. Muscles tense up. The mind is overworking and the spirit is repressed and suppressed.

Outside: Body is tired and worn out, posture is slumped.

Reaction: To be unmotivated (have no interest or enthusiasm), to be fatigued.

Root Cause: Sadness.

DESPAIR

Meaning: A state of mind where you feel there is nothing you can do to improve a difficult situation.

Purpose: To help you to find strength within and surrender to a higher power.
Feeling: Helpless, hopeless, powerless.

WHAT HAPPENS TO THE BODY?

Inside: The anterior cingulate cortex, which is the part of the brain responsible for regulating emotions and processing pain, is activated. The sympathetic nervous system, which is responsible for the fight-or-flight response, is activated. The stress hormone cortisol – which is responsible for mood, motivation and emotions and for alerting or shutting down bodily functions, such as the digestive, immune and reproductive systems – is released into the bloodstream. Heart rate increases. Rapid breathing. Blood pressure increases. Muscles contract. Blood vessels constrict.
Outside: Body is tensed.
Reaction: To resist, to struggle.
Root Cause: Fear, sadness.

DISAPPOINTED

Meaning: A state of mind that makes you feel let down because something or someone has failed to meet your expectations and not given you what you wanted.
Purpose: To help you be aware that you were expecting an outcome and it has not happened; to help you be aware something you wanted did not go your way.
Feeling: Displeased, dissatisfied, unhappy.

WHAT HAPPENS TO THE BODY?

Inside: The amygdala, which is the part of the brain responsible for assessing the environment, detects disappointment and alerts the hippocampus. The hippocampus, which is responsible for storing episodic memories, will trigger a past experience to help your body to respond to a similar situation. The hypothalamus, which is responsible for releasing hormones, is alerted and sends a message to the adrenal glands. The adrenal glands, which are responsible for stress hormones, release cortisol. Cortisol, which helps the body respond to stress, releases energy and shuts down other body functions, such as the digestive, immune and reproductive systems. Digestion and breathing become irregular. Blood vessels constrict. Blood pressure increases. Muscles tense. Mood is impacted. Body is low on energy.

Outside: Body withdraws, posture slumps.

Reaction: To lose faith.

Root Cause: Sadness.

DISCONNECTED

Meaning: A mental state of mind and being where you feel no connection with anything or anyone in your life or with life itself.

Purpose: To help you be aware you have lost connection to your whole self; to help you to heal, and release and find new ways to reconnect back to yourself.

Feeling: Confused, isolated, lonely.

WHAT HAPPENS TO THE BODY?

Inside: The stress hormone cortisol – which is responsible for mood, motivation and emotions and for alerting or shutting down body functions such as the digestive, immune, and reproductive systems – is activated. The circulatory system, which pumps blood to your heart, is unregulated. Blood pressure rises.

Outside: Body withdraws.

Reaction: To withdraw.

Root Cause: Sadness.

DISCONTENT

Meaning: A state of mind and being where you feel you are not getting what you want or need in life.

Purpose: To help you to be aware that you do not feel whole.

Feeling: Dissatisfaction, unhappy, unfulfilled.

WHAT HAPPENS TO THE BODY?

Inside: The amygdala, which is the part of the brain responsible for processing emotion and behaviour and assessing the environment, detects unhappiness and alerts the hippocampus. The hippocampus, which is responsible for storing episodic memories, triggers a past experience to help your body respond to a similar situation. The parasympathetic nervous system, which is responsible for slowing heart rate and increasing gland activity, is activated. Heartbeat decreases. Breath decreases. Blood vessels constrict. Blood pressure increases. Muscles tense. Blood flow decreases.

Outside: Posture is slumped.

Reaction: To complain.

Root Cause: Sadness.

DISCOURAGED

Meaning: A state of mind and being that makes you feel as if your spirit is being dampened by something or someone.

Purpose: To help you to surrender to the current way and find a new way.

Feeling: Dismay, disheartened, disappointed, hopeless.

WHAT HAPPENS TO THE BODY?

Inside: The amygdala, which is the part of the brain responsible for assessing the environment, detects a sense of discouragement and alerts the hippocampus. The hippocampus, which stores episodic memories, triggers a past experience to help your body to respond to a similar situation. The hypothalamus, which is the part of the brain responsible for releasing hormones, is alerted. The stress hormone cortisol, which helps the body respond to stress, releases energy and shuts down other body functions such as the digestive, immune and reproductive systems. Digestion and breathing become irregular. Blood vessels constrict. Blood pressure increases. Muscles tense.

Outside: Posture is slumped.

Reaction: To lose faith, to give up (stop making an effort).

Root Cause: Sadness.

DISGUST

Meaning: A state of mind and being where you have a strong feeling aroused by something unpleasant or offensive.

Purpose: To make you aware that you severely dislike something.

Feeling: Repulsed, unhappy.

WHAT HAPPENS TO THE BODY?

Inside: The cerebral cortex, which is the part of the brain responsible for perception, senses disgust. The insula, which is the part of the brain responsible for pain and perception, receives the message of disgust. The autonomic nervous system which has a direct role in the physical response to stress, digestion, respiratory rate and pupillary response, is triggered. Heartbeat slows. Breathing is irregular.

Outside: A crumpled facial expression, body shivers, body withdraws.

Reaction: To reject, to withdraw.

Root Cause: Fear.

DISSATISFIED

Meaning: A state of mind and being that causes a feeling that something is not as good as it should be.

Purpose: To help you be aware that an outcome has not turned out as expected.

Feeling: Unhappy, discontent, disappointed.

WHAT HAPPENS TO THE BODY?

Inside: The amygdala, which is the part of the brain responsible for assessing the environment, detects dissatisfaction and alerts the hippocampus. The hippocampus, which is the part of the brain responsible for storing episodic memories, triggers a past experience to help your body to respond to a similar situation. The hypothalamus, which is the part of the brain responsible for releasing hormones, is alerted and sends a message to the adrenal glands. The adrenal glands, which are responsible for stress hormones, releases cortisol. Cortisol, which helps the body respond to stress, releases energy and shuts down other functions such as the digestive, immune and reproductive systems. Digestion and breathing become irregular. Blood vessels constrict. Blood pressure increases. Muscles tense.

Outside: Posture slumps.

Reaction: To criticize.

Root Cause: Fear, sadness.

DISTURBED

Meaning: A state of mind and being where a normal pattern or function is disrupted.

Purpose: To help you step out of yourself and be aware of something or someone.

Feeling: Annoyed, distressed, irritated, stressed.

WHAT HAPPENS TO THE BODY?

Inside: The amygdala, which is the part of the brain that is responsible for emotions and the assessment of your environment, detects a sense of disturbance. The prefrontal cortex, which is responsible for decision-making, sends a message to the hypothalamus. The hypothalamus, which is responsible for releasing hormones and actioning the fight-or-flight response, is activated. The hormone adrenalin, which alerts your brain and body for action, is released into the bloodstream. The stress hormone cortisol, which helps the body respond to stress and shuts down other body functions such as the digestive, immune and reproductive systems, functions that get in the way (such as the digestive, immune and reproductive systems), is released into the bloodstream. Heart rate increases. Breathing is rapid. The digestive, immune and reproductive systems are irregular.

Outside: Pupils dilate, senses heighten, body is disrupted.

Reaction: To be unsettled.

Root cause: Fear, sadness.

DISTRAUGHT

Meaning: A state of mind and being where you are feeling being deeply upset about something.

Purpose: To help you be aware that something bad has happened.

Feeling: Unhappy, distressed.

WHAT HAPPENS TO THE BODY?

Inside: The amygdala, which is the part of the brain responsible for receiving incoming messages, receives a message that something bad has happened. The sympathetic nervous system, which is responsible for preparing the body for fight and flight, is activated. The lachrymal gland, which produces tears, is triggered. Heart rate and breathing are irregular. Muscles contract.

Outside: Face and body crumples.

Reaction: To cry.

Root Cause: Fear, sadness.

DOUBTFUL

Meaning: A state of mind and being that makes you feel uncertain.

Purpose: To help you to connect to your intuition and find power within.

Feeling: Confused.

WHAT HAPPENS TO THE BODY?

Inside: The prefrontal cortex – the part of the brain that detects our sense of self, our value system, and is responsible for our self-control – fires messages back and forth to the amygdala. The amygdala, which is the emotional centre of the brain, receives the messages as a potential threat and sends a warning to the hypothalamus. The hypothalamus, which is the part of the brain responsible for releasing hormones and actioning the flight-or-fight response, sends a message to the body to prepare for a threat. The steroid hormone cortisol, which deals with stress and shuts down other body functions not needed (such as the immune and reproductive systems or growth), is activated and released into the bloodstream. Breathing is restricted. Blood flow is reduced. Muscles tense and tighten.

Outside: Body is restless.

Reaction: To be cautious.

Root Cause: Fear.

DREAD

Meaning: A state of mind and being where you feel scared about something that will happen.

Purpose: To help you be aware that you are scared of something and need to search for a way to get through it.

Feeling: Anxious, frightened, scared, worried.

WHAT HAPPENS TO THE BODY?

Inside: The amygdala, which is the part of your brain responsible for activating the fight-or-flight response, receives a message of potential danger; it sends a signal to the hypothalamus, which triggers a fight-or-flight response. The perception of threat activates the sympathetic nervous system and triggers an acute stress response that prepares the body to fight or flight. Heartbeat speeds up. The stress hormones adrenalin and cortisol are released into the bloodstream.

Outside: Body is uptight and tense

Reaction: To fight, to freeze or to flee (flight).

Root Cause: Fear.

EMBARRASSED

Meaning: A state of mind and being that makes you feel bad because something doesn't feel right to you.

Purpose: To help you be aware and go within and find your self-worth.

Feeling: Ashamed.

WHAT HAPPENS TO THE BODY?

Inside: The anterior cingulate cortex, which is the part of the brain responsible for emotional pain, attention and decision-making, detects a threatening situation. The hypothalamus, which is the part of the brain that actions the fight-or-flight response and the release of hormones, is instantly activated.

Dictionary

The hormone adrenalin, which keeps your body alert and energized, receives a message from the brain that a stressful situation is taking place and is released into the bloodstream. The capillaries that carry your blood widen, which causes the blood to rush to the surface of your skin. Heart rate and breathing increase. Muscles tense.

Outside: Eyes divert, skin blushes, body shrinks.

Reaction: To withdraw.

Root Cause: Fear.

EMPTY

Meaning: A state of mind or being where you feel like you are empty on the inside.

Purpose: To help you be aware that you need to find meaning in your life.

Feeling: Unfulfilled.

WHAT HAPPENS TO THE BODY?

Inside: The amygdala, which is the part of the brain that is responsible for assessing the environment. detects dissatisfaction and alerts the hippocampus. The hippocampus. which is the part of the brain responsible for storing episodic memories, triggers a past experience to help your body respond to a similar situation. The hypothalamus, which is the part of the brain responsible for releasing hormones, is alerted. The stress hormone cortisol, which helps the body respond to stress, releases energy and shuts down other body functions (such as the digestive, immune and reproductive systems). Digestion and breathing become irregular. Blood vessels constrict. Blood pressure increases. Muscles tense.

Outside: To withdraw.

Reaction: To be on autopilot (act without thinking or feeling).

Root Cause: Sadness.

ENVIOUS

Meaning: A state of mind and being that makes you feel bad because you wish you had what another person has.

Purpose: To make you aware that you feel you are missing or lacking something in life.

Feeling: Angry, inadequate, jealous, unfulfilled, unhappy. Envy can also lead to low self-esteem.

WHAT HAPPENS TO THE BODY?

Inside: The front lobe, which is the part of your brain responsible for analysing social situations and processing information before making a judgement, is activated. The amygdala, which is the part of the brain responsible for assessing the environment, detects dissatisfaction and alerts the hippocampus. The hippocampus, which is responsible for storing episodic memories, triggers a past experience to help your body to respond to a similar situation. The hypothalamus, which is responsible for releasing hormones, is alerted and sends a message to the adrenal glands. The adrenal glands, which are responsible for stress hormones, release cortisol. Cortisol, which helps the body respond to stress, releases energy. Heartbeat increases. Rapid breathing. Blood pressure rises. Muscles tense.

Outside: Body becomes tense and tight.

Reaction: To fight or flee (take flight).

Root Cause: Fear.

FOOLISH

Meaning: A state of mind and being that makes you feel like you did not make the right choice.

Purpose: To make you aware that something happened and it did not help you in life.

Feeling: Hurt, embarrassed.

WHAT HAPPENS TO THE BODY?

Inside: The anterior cingulate cortex, which is the part of the brain responsible for emotional pain, attention and decision-making, detects a threatening situation. The hypothalamus, which is the part of the brain that actions the fight-or-flight response and the release of hormones, is instantly activated. The hormone adrenalin, which keeps your body alert and energized, receives a message from the brain that a stressful situation is taking place and is released into the bloodstream. The capillaries that carry your blood widen and cause the blood to rush to the surface of your skin. Heart rate and breathing are increased. Muscles tense.

Outside: Body withdraws.

Reaction: To self-doubt, to lose confidence.

Root Cause: Fear.

FRIGHTENED

Meaning: A state of mind and being that makes you scared.

Purpose: To make you aware that you are not feeling safe.

Feeling: Afraid, anxious, worried.

WHAT HAPPENS TO THE BODY?

Inside: The amygdala, which is the part of your brain responsible for activating the fight-or-flight response, receives a message of potential danger, so it sends a signal to the hypothalamus, which triggers the fight-or-flight response The perception of threat activates the sympathetic nervous system, and triggers an acute stress response that prepares the body for fight or flight. Heartbeat speeds up. The stress hormones adrenalin and cortisol are released into the bloodstream. Blood vessels constrict. Muscles tense. Breathing quickens.

Outside: Eyes widen, pupils dilate, body is on high alert.
Reaction: To fight, freeze or take flight.
Root Cause: Fear.

FRUSTRATED

Meaning: A state of mind and being that makes you feel an emotional pain because you cannot change or achieve something, and this is stopping you from getting what you want.

Purpose: To help you be aware that you are in a situation you are struggling to change or you are being denied or blocked; to help you be aware a goal is not being achieved, and to help you surrender and find a new way to approach this.

Feeling: Angry, annoyed, irritated, dissatisfied, disappointed, unfulfilled, unhappy, powerless. Frustration can lead to deeper places of negative states, and distort your worldview.

WHAT HAPPENS TO THE BODY?

Inside: The amygdala, which is the part of the brain responsible for receiving incoming messages from your senses, detects frustration and sends a message to the hypothalamus. The hypothalamus is connected to the nervous system and the fight-or-flight trigger is activated. The sympathetic nervous system releases hormones into the bloodstream. The stress hormone cortisol, which pushes the body into action to combat stress, is released. Adrenalin, which distributes blood away from the heart and to muscles in readiness for action, is released. The digestive, immune and reproductive systems slow down and are suppressed. Heart rate speeds up. Rapid breathing. Blood pressure rises. Blood vessels constrict. Muscles tighten and tense.

Outside: Body is tense.
Reaction: To be distressed.
Root Cause: Fear.

FURIOUS

Meaning: An emotional state of mind and being where you are feeling full of fury.

Purpose: To help give you strength to make a change and drive you forward.

Feeling: Angry.

WHAT HAPPENS TO THE BODY?

Inside: The amygdala, which is the emotional centre of the brain and responsible for perception and assessment, recognizes a threat and sends a message to the hypothalamus. The hypothalamus, which is responsible for releasing hormones actioning the fight-or-flight response, is activated. The hormone adrenalin, which keeps your body alert and energized, receives a message from the brain that a stressful situation is taking place and is released into the bloodstream. The sympathetic nervous system, which is responsible for stimulating the body's fight-or-flight response, is activated. The stress hormone cortisol – which is responsible for mood, motivation and emotions and alerting or shutting down body functions such as the digestive, immune and reproductive systems and growth processes – is activated. The hormone noradrenaline, which mobilizes the brain and body for action, increases the heart rate and helps to shift blood flow towards muscles, is activated. Breathing increases. Muscles contract. Blood vessels constrict.

Outside: Pupils dilate, senses heighten, body is energized.

Reaction: To act and react.

Root cause: Fear, sadness.

GRIEF

Meaning: A mental state of mind and being where you experience a deep emotional loss and pain because someone or something that you had a bond with, attachment to or affection for has gone from your life.

Purpose: To help you be aware of the loss, and to help you move through the loss.

Feeling: Anger, confused, hurt, isolated, guilt, heartbroken, lonely, rage, regret, resentment, shock, worry, vulnerable.

WHAT HAPPENS TO THE BODY?

Inside: The somatosensory cortex, which is the part of the brain that receives and processes sensory information and feels sensations, is activated. The anterior insula, which is the part of the brain responsible for sensory signals and feeling sensations, is activated. The anterior cingulate cortex, which is the part of the brain responsible for regulating emotions and processing the perception of pain, is activated. The hippocampus, which is the part of the brain responsible for storing your life stories, memories and associations, is activated. The amygdala, which is the part of the brain responsible for fear and triggering the fight-or-flight response, becomes over-activated. The nervous system, which keeps your body in a homeostasis state and balances the body, becomes irregular. The parasympathetic nervous system, which releases the stress hormones cortisol and adrenalin into your bloodstream, is irregular. The sympathetic nervous system, which conserves energy in your body and sets your body for rest, is underactive or overactive. The circulatory system, which circulates blood to your heart and brain and throughout your body, becomes irregular. Your immune and digestive systems become irregular. Heart rate is irregular. Breathing is irregular. Blood pressure rises. Muscles tense.

Outside: Headache, tight chest, shortness of breath, dizziness, nausea, stomach pain, lack of appetite.

Dictionary

Reaction: To be bereft, to mourn, to yearn.
Root Cause: Sadness.

GRIEF-STRICKEN
Meaning: A state of mind and being where you are overwhelmed by a huge amount of grief.
Purpose: To help you be aware that a huge loss and change has occurred, which you did not expect or are not ready for.
Feeling: Grief, heartbroken; broken heart syndrome is a temporary heart condition that's often brought on by stressful situations and extreme emotions.

WHAT HAPPENS TO THE BODY?
Inside: The limbic system, which is the part of the brain responsible for processing emotions, deactivates. The amygdala, which is part of the limbic system and responsible for processing information for flight or flight, deactivates. The thalamus, which is the part of the brain responsible for feelings through temperature, touch, pain and pleasure, deactivates. The hippocampus, which is the part of the brain responsible for storing life experiences and how they feel in the body, deactivates. The circulatory system, which helps blood flow through the body and pumps oxygen towards the heart and brain, decreases. Blood flow severely decreases. Blood pressure severely decreases. Brain lacks blood flow and oxygen. The respiratory system, which absorbs oxygen through the nose, mouth and lungs, over-activates. Heart rate drops. Rapid breathing. Blood flow decreases. Muscles severely tense. Irregular heartbeat. Low blood pressure. Brain becomes foggy.
External: Chest pain, shortness of breath.
Outside: To break down (collapse emotionally, physically and/ or spiritually), to be devastated.
Root Cause: Sadness.

Guilty

Meaning: A state of mind and being that makes you feel as if you are doing something wrong.

Purpose: To help you be aware of your actions and reactions and your whole self.

Feeling: Shame. Guilt can lead you deeper into other negative states and towards addiction-related behaviour.

What happens to the body?

Inside: The prefrontal cortex, which is the part of the brain responsible for attention and predicting consequences of actions, is activated. The amygdala, which is the part of the brain responsible for processing emotions and behaviour, is activated. The insula, which is part of the brain responsible for perception and pain, is activated. The sympathetic nervous system, which is responsible for fight and flight, is activated. The pituitary gland, which releases stress hormones, is activated. The stress hormone cortisol, which is responsible for mood, motivation and emotions and alerting and shutting down body functions (such as the digestive, immune and reproductive systems), is released into the bloodstream. Heart rate is increased. Blood pressure is increased. Breath is irregular. Muscles constrict.

Outside: Body is restless.

Reaction: To overcompensate.

Root cause: Fear.

Hate

Meaning: A state of mind and being that makes you feel a deep and intense dislike towards someone or something.

Purpose: To help you protect yourself and your loved ones from danger and harm.

Feeling: Animosity, anger, disgust, rage, resentment

Dictionary

What happens to the body?

Inside: The frontal lobe, which is the part of the brain responsible for personality, problem-solving and behaviour, deactivates. The premotor cortex, which is the part of the brain responsible for planning and execution of motion and preparing the body muscle for movement, is activated. The putamen, which is the part of the brain that helps control activity and movement, is activated. The insula, which is the part of the brain responsible for processing emotional experience and for the perception of disgust, is activated. The autonomic nervous system triggers the fight-or-flight response and releases the stress hormones cortisol and adrenalin into the bloodstream. Heart rate speeds up, rapid breathing. Blood pressure rises. Blood vessels constrict. Muscles tighten and tense.

Outside: Eyes constrict, body is uptight and rigid.

Reaction: To attack, to reject, to distrust, to withdraw.

Root Cause: Fear.

Heartbroken

Meaning: A state of mind and being that makes you feel like you are suffering from an intense emotional and physical pain due to the loss of someone or something.

Purpose: To make you aware that you have lost someone or something you love.

Feeling: Anguish, distress, hurt, sorrow, grief; broken heart syndrome is a temporary heart condition that is often brought on by hurt, and that pain leads to other stressful situations and extremely painful emotions.

What happens to the body?

Inside: The anterior insula, which is the part of the brain responsible for sensory signals and feeling sensations, is activated. The anterior cingulate cortex, which is the part of the brain responsible for regulating emotions and processing the perception of pain, is activated. The amygdala, which is the part of the brain responsible for triggering fight or flight, is activated. The adrenal cortex, which is responsible for releasing the stress hormone cortisol into the bloodstream, is activated. Cortisol is released into the bloodstream. The circulatory system, which circulates blood to your heart and brain and throughout your body, becomes irregular. Your immune and digestive systems become irregular. Heart rate decreases. Muscles contract.

Outside: Angina, shortness of breath.

Reaction: To be withdrawn or disoriented.

Root Cause: Sadness.

HELPLESS

Meaning: A state of mind where you feel you are unable to do anything to help yourself or anyone else.

Purpose: To help you to surrender to yourself as a whole and to find power from within. Feeling helpless is also a chance for you to reconnect and unite to others and to open yourself up to seeing a new way.

Feeling: Hopeless, powerless.

WHAT HAPPENS TO THE BODY?

Inside: The cerebral cortex, which is the part of the brain responsible for perception, thinking, language and voluntary action, becomes overactivate. The amygdala, which is responsible for processing emotions, becomes overactivate. The thalamus, which is responsible for triggering emotions connected to past events, is activated. The somatosensory cortex, which is the part of the brain that receives and processes sensory information from the entire body, is activated. Homeostatic regulation, which controls the balance of cells in your body, gets disrupted. The endocrine system, which is responsible for releasing hormones into the bloodstream and works in balance with the immune system and nervous system, becomes unregulated. The cardiovascular system, which pumps blood to the heart and brain, is disrupted. The respiratory system, which helps you to breathe, is disrupted. Heart rate and breathing are irregular. Muscles tighten and constrict. Blood flow is restricted.

Outside: Body is restless.

Reaction: To fight or take flight.

Root Cause: Fear, sadness.

HOMESICK

Meaning: A state of mind and being where you are longing and yearning for a place you call home because you feel so far away from it.

Purpose: To help you be aware that you are longing to be back in a place of comfort or familiarity; to help you remember a place where you came from – your roots.

Feeling: Anxious, depressed, grief, insecure, nostalgic, unhappy, uncomfortable, uneasy.

WHAT HAPPENS TO THE BODY?

Inside: The hippocampus, which is the part of the brain responsible for repeating episodic memories, are activated. The amygdala, which is responsible for processing emotions, becomes overactivate. The thalamus, which is responsible for triggering emotions related to past events, is activated. The somatosensory cortex, which is a part of the brain that receives and processes sensory information from the entire body, is activated. Homeostatic regulation, which controls the balance of cells in your body, gets disrupted. The endocrine system, which releases hormones into the bloodstream and works in balance with the immune system and nervous system, is disrupted. The cardiovascular system, which pumps blood to the heart and brain, is disrupted. The respiratory system, which is responsible for helping you to breathe, is disrupted. Heart rate and breathing are irregular. Muscles tighten and constrict. Blood flow is restricted.

Outside: Body is restless.

Reaction: To yearn.

Root Cause: Fear, sadness.

HOPELESS

Meaning: A state of mind and being where you feel events, situations and circumstances in your life are not going well and will not turn out for the best.

Purpose: To make you aware that you have lost hope and see no way out for help.

Feeling: Unhappy, powerless.

WHAT HAPPENS TO THE BODY?

Inside: The amygdala, which is the part of the brain responsible for processing emotions, is activated. The hippocampus, which is part of the brain responsible for repeating life memories, is activated. The thalamus, which is responsible for triggering emotions connected to past events, is activated. The parasympathetic nervous system, which is responsible for slowing the heart rate and increasing gland activity, is activated. The feel-good chemicals dopamine and serotonin, which are responsible for wellbeing and balancing mood, decrease. Heartbeat slows. Breathing slows. Blood vessels constrict. Blood pressure increases. Muscles tense. Blood flow decreases.

Outside: Body slumps.

Reaction: To mope (wander aimlessly).
Root Cause: Sadness.

Hostile
Meaning: A state of mind and being where you feel opposed to what is happening.
Purpose: To make you aware that something in your life is not going your way.
Feeling: Angry, hate.
What happens to the body?
Inside: The amygdala, which is the part of the brain responsible for receiving incoming messages, receives a message of threat. The anterior cingulate cortex, which is responsible for regulating emotions and processing pain, is activated. The autonomic nervous system, which triggers the fight-or-flight response and releases the stress hormones cortisol and adrenalin into the bloodstream, is activated. Heart rate speeds up. Rapid breathing. Blood pressure rises. Blood vessels constrict. Muscles tense.
Outside: Body is tense.
Reaction: To resist.
Root Cause: Fear.

Humiliated
Meaning: An emotional state of mind and being where you feel your status is reduced to nothing.
Purpose: To help you to step into your whole self and overcome the illusion of status.
Feeling: Shame, embarrassed. (A fear of being humiliated can lead to social phobia – a fear of being watched and judged by others. This can lead to anxiety and other negative states that are hard to move away from.)

WHAT HAPPENS TO THE BODY?

Inside: The amygdala, which is the part of the brain responsible for receiving incoming messages, receives a message of threat and danger and sends a message to the hypothalamus, which immediately triggers the fight-or-flight response. The sympathetic nervous system, which prepares the body for fight and flight, is activated. The stress hormone cortisol, which increases energy, is released into the bloodstream. Adrenalin, which distributes blood to muscles, is released. Heart rate speeds up. Rapid breathing. Blood pressure rises. Blood vessels constrict. Muscles tense.

Outside: Skin is flushed, body is tense.

Reaction: To fight or take flight.

Root Cause: Fear.

HURT

Meaning: A state of mind and being that creates a deep emotional pain within.

Purpose: To help you be aware that you are being devalued.

Feeling: Unhappy, distressed, uncomfortable, restless. (Hurt is felt when you feel abandoned, rejected, ignored, criticized, betrayed, maliciously teased, underappreciated, undervalued. There are different areas of pain when hurt: physical pain, which is created through damage to your body; social pain, which is created through interacting with others; and psychological pain, which is created through the mind.)

WHAT HAPPENS TO THE BODY?

Inside: The anterior insula, which is the part of the brain responsible for feeling sensations in the body, is activated. The anterior cingulate cortex, which is the part of the brain responsible for regulating emotions and processing pain, is

activated. The somatosensory cortex, which is a part of the brain that receives and processes sensory information that impacts the entire body, is activated. The sympathetic nervous system, which prepares the body's fight-or-flight response, is activated. The stress hormone cortisol – which is responsible for mood, motivation and emotions and for alerting or shutting down body functions, such as the digestive, immune and reproductive systems – is released into the bloodstream. Heart rate increases. Rapid breathing. Blood pressure increases. Muscles contract. Blood vessels constrict.
Outside: Body withdraws.
Reaction: To defend, to protect.
Root Cause: Sadness.

Impatient
Meaning: A state of mind and being where you feel rushed because you need to get somewhere and you feel like something is stopping you from where you want or need to be.
Purpose: To help you be aware that you are not where you want to be.
Feeling: Irritated.
What happens to the body?
Inside: The amygdala, which is the part of the brain responsible for receiving incoming messages from your senses, detects threat or danger and sends a message to the hypothalamus. The hypothalamus is connected to the nervous system and triggers the fight-or-flight response. The sympathetic nervous system, which releases hormones into the bloodstream, is activated. The stress hormone cortisol, which pushes the body into action to combat stress, is released into the bloodstream. Adrenalin, which distributes blood away from the heart and to muscles ready for action, is released. The digestive, immune and

reproductive systems slow down and are suppressed. Heart rate speeds up. Rapid breathing. Blood pressure rises. Blood vessels constrict. Muscles tense.

Outside: Body is restless.

Reaction: To push.

Root Cause: Fear.

INADEQUATE

Meaning: A state of mind and being where you feel a strong sense that you are not good enough.

Purpose: To help you be aware that something or someone is making you feel less than you are; to help you find your self-worth and connect to yourself as a whole.

Feeling: Insecure.

WHAT HAPPENS TO THE BODY?

Inside: The hippocampus, which is the part of the brain responsible for repeating life memories, is activated. The amygdala, which is responsible for processing emotions, becomes over activated. The thalamus, which is responsible for triggering emotions connected to past events, is activated. The somatosensory cortex, which is the part of the brain that receives and processes sensory information from the entire body, is activated. Homeostatic regulation, which controls the balance of cells in your body, is disrupted. The endocrine system, which releases hormones into the bloodstream and works in balance with the immune system and nervous system, is disrupted. The cardiovascular system, which pumps blood to the heart and brain, is disrupted. The respiratory system, which helps you breathe, is disrupted. Heart rate and breathing is Irregular. Muscles tense. Blood flow is restricted.

Outside: Body is off balance.

Rection: To fight or take flight.
Root Cause: Fear, sadness.

INFERIOR

Meaning: A state of mind and being that makes you feel you are lower in rank, status or quality to another.

Purpose: To help you be aware that you feel less than and are not connected to your whole self or are not seeing your self-worth.

Feeling: Insecure, inadequate. (A repeated feeling of inferiority can lead to low self-esteem – when you start to lose confidence in who you are and what you can do in life.)

WHAT HAPPENS TO THE BODY?

Inside: The hippocampus, which is the part of the brain responsible for repeating life memories, is activated. The amygdala, which is responsible for processing emotions, becomes overactivate. The thalamus, which is responsible for triggering emotions connected to past events, is activated. The somatosensory cortex, which is a part of the brain that receives and processes sensory information from the entire body, is activated. Homeostatic regulation, which controls the balance of cells in your body, gets disrupted. The endocrine system, which releases hormones into the bloodstream and works in balance with the immune system and nervous system, is disrupted. The cardiovascular system, which pumps blood to the heart and brain, is disrupted. The respiratory system, which helping you to breathe, is disrupted. Heart rate and breathing are irregular. Muscles tense. Blood flow is restricted.

Outside: Body is off balance.

Reaction: To withdraw.

Root Cause: Fear.

INSECURE

Meaning: A state of mind and being that gives you a feeling that you are in a position that is not firm or fixed and can easily give way or break.

Purpose: To help you be aware that you do not feel safe or trust where you are.

Feeling: Anxious, uneasy. (A constant feeling of insecurity can lead you to always feeling fear.)

WHAT HAPPENS TO THE BODY?

Inside: The amygdala, which is the part of the brain responsible for receiving incoming messages from your senses, detects threat or danger and sends a message to the hypothalamus. The hypothalamus, which is the part of the brain connected to the nervous system and which triggers the fight-or-flight response, is activated. The sympathetic nervous system, which releases stress hormones into the bloodstream and triggers fight and flight, is activated. The stress hormone cortisol, which pushes the body into action to combat stress, is released. Adrenalin, which distributes blood away from the heart and towards muscles in readiness for action, is activated. Heart rate speeds up. Rapid breathing. Blood pressure rises. Blood vessels constrict, muscles tense.

Outside: Body tenses.

Reaction: To fight or take flight.

Root Cause: Fear.

INSULTED

Meaning: A state of mind and being that gives you the feeling of being offended by something said and done.

Purpose: To help you be aware that you are allowing something or someone to impact how you feel about yourself.

Feeling: Annoyed, angry, hurt, upset.

Dictionary

What happens to the body?

Inside: The amygdala, which is the part of the brain responsible for receiving incoming messages, receives a message of threat and danger and sends a message to the hypothalamus, which immediately triggers the fight-or-flight response. The somatosensory cortex, which is the part of the brain that receives and processes information from your senses, is activated. The sympathetic nervous system, which is responsible for preparing the body for fight and flight, is activated. The stress hormone cortisol, which increases energy, is released into the bloodstream. Adrenalin, which distributes blood to the muscles, is released. Heart rate speeds up. Rapid breathing. Blood pressure rises. Blood vessels constrict. Muscles tense.
Outside: Body tenses.
Reaction: To defend.
Root cause: Fear.

Irritated

Meaning: A state of mind and being where you feel gradual arousal and a build-up of uncomfortable feelings.
Purpose: To make you aware that you are not comfortable with where you are or what is happening at that moment.
Feeling: Anger, annoyed, impatience, unhappy. (Mild irritation can lead to deeper negative states.)

What happens to the body?

Inside: The amygdala, which is the part of the brain responsible for receiving incoming messages from your senses, detects irritation and sends a message to the hypothalamus. The hypothalamus, which is connected to the nervous system, triggers the fight-or-flight response. The sympathetic nervous system, which releases hormones into the bloodstream, is activated. The stress hormone cortisol, which pushes the body into action to combat stress, is released into the bloodstream. Adrenalin, which distributes blood away from the heart and towards muscles in readiness for action, is released. The digestive, immune and reproductive systems slow down. Heart rate speeds up. Rapid breathing. Blood pressure rises. Blood vessels constrict. Muscles tense.

Outside: Body is restless.

Reaction: To snap.

Root cause: Fear, sadness.

ISOLATED

Meaning: A state of mind and being where you feel a strong sense that you are completely alone and separate – unable to relate or connect with anything or anyone.

Purpose: To help you to connect to your whole self, inside and out, for inner growth and development.

Feeling: Anxious, confused, lonely, insecure, frightened.

WHAT HAPPENS TO THE BODY?

Inside: The amygdala, which is the part of the brain responsible for processing emotion and behaviour and assessing the environment, detects loneliness and alerts the hippocampus. The hippocampus, which is the part of the brain responsible for storing life memories, triggers a past experience to help your body respond to a similar situation. The endocrine system, which releases hormones into the bloodstream and works in balance with the immune and nervous systems, is disrupted. The stress hormones cortisol and adrenalin are released into the bloodstream. The cardiovascular system, which pumps blood to the heart and brain, is disrupted. The respiratory system, which helps you breathe, is disrupted. Heart rate and breathing are irregular. Muscles tighten. Blood flow is restricted.

External: Body is restless.
Outside: To withdraw.
Root Cause: Fear, sadness.

JEALOUS
Meaning: A state of mind and being where you feel resentment towards someone because of their achievements, possessions or perceived advantages.
Purpose: To help you be aware that you feel threatened by something or someone and do not feel good enough where you are. (Beware: jealousy can cause you to move away from stepping inside your whole self and finding your power.)
Feeling: Angry, inadequate, insecure.
WHAT HAPPENS TO THE BODY?
Inside: The frontal lobe, which is the part of your brain responsible for analysing social situations and processing information before making a judgement, is activated. The amygdala, which is the part of the brain responsible for receiving incoming messages, receives a message of threat and danger and sends a message to the hypothalamus, which immediately triggers the fight-or-flight response. The sympathetic nervous system, which prepares the body for fight and flight, is activated. The stress hormone cortisol, which increases energy in the bloodstream. is released. Adrenalin, which distributes blood to muscles, is released. Heart rate speeds up. Rapid breathing. Blood pressure rises. Blood vessels constrict. Muscles tense. Peripheral vision is lost, causing tunnel vision. Hearing decreases.
Outside: Body tenses.
Reaction: To fight or take flight.
Root Cause: Fear.

LONELY

Meaning: A mental state of mind and being where you feel completely alone, without any form of connection or any companions to connect with.

Purpose: To help you connect to your whole self; to help you connect to life. (In life, it is normal to feel lonely on your journey. You are the only one to experience life from your position and perspective, and in your body and with your feelings. Remember, you are not alone in loneliness. The way to move through loneliness is to understand this and find someone to talk to.)

Feeling: Isolated, anxious, angry, depressed.

WHAT HAPPENS TO THE BODY?

Inside: The amygdala, which is the part of the brain responsible for processing emotion and behaviour and assessing the environment, detects a sense of being and alerts the hippocampus. The hippocampus, which is responsible for storing episodic memories, triggers a past experience to help your body respond to a similar situation. The parasympathetic nervous system, which slows the heart rate and increases gland activity, is activated. Heartbeat slows. Breathing slows. Blood vessels constrict. Blood pressure increases. Muscles tense. Blood flow decreases.

Outside: Body withdraws.

Reaction: To be angry, to cry, to be confused.

Root Cause: Sadness.

LOST

Meaning: A mental state of mind and being where you do not know where you are.

Feeling: Confused, lonely.

Purpose: To help you be aware you have wandered far away from yourself.

What happens to the body?

Inside: The amygdala, which is the part of the brain responsible for receiving incoming messages, receives a message of threat and danger and sends a message to the hypothalamus, which immediately triggers the fight-or-flight response. The sympathetic nervous system, which is prepares the body for fight and flight, is activated. The stress hormone cortisol, which increases energy in the bloodstream, is released. Adrenalin, which distributes blood to muscles, is released. Noradrenaline, which is responsible for alertness and mobilizing the brain and body for action, is released. The immune, digestive and reproductive systems are suppressed or shut down. Heart rate speeds up. Rapid breathing. Muscles tense.

Outside: Body is restless.

Reaction: To search.

Root Cause: Fear.

Miserable

Meaning: A state of mind and being where you feel you are leading an uncomfortable existence.

Purpose: To help you be aware that you do not like what is happening or where you are.

Feeling: Unhappy.

What happens to the body?

Inside: The amygdala, which is the part of the brain responsible for processing emotion and behaviour and assessing the environment, detects misery and alerts the hippocampus. The hippocampus, which is responsible for storing episodic memories, triggers a past experience to help your body respond to a similar situation. The parasympathetic nervous system, which slows the heart rate and increases gland activity, is activated. Heartbeat speeds up. Breathing slows. Blood vessels constrict. Blood pressure increases. Muscles tense. Blood flow decreases.

Outside: Body slumps.

Reaction: To complain.

Root Cause: Sadness.

NOSTALGIC

Meaning: A state of mind where you find yourself returning to a former time in your life; can be a positive or negative experience depending on how you view it.

Purpose: To help you to be aware that time is passing by and to connect with life.

Feeling: Unhappy.

WHAT HAPPENS TO THE BODY?

Inside: The hippocampus, which is part of the brain responsible for storing your life memory, is activated. The parasympathetic nervous system, which slows the heart rate and increases gland activity, is activated. The hormone acetylcholine, responsible for dilating blood vessels and increasing bodily secretions, is released. Heartbeat slows. Breathing slows. Blood vessels constrict. Blood pressure increases. Muscles tense. Blood flow decreases.

Outside: Body slumps.

Reaction: To desire, to yearn.

Root Cause: Sadness.

NERVOUS

Meaning: A state of mind and being where you are not comfortable or relaxed with what is happening at that moment or in the future.

Purpose: To help you be aware that you are experiencing or will soon experience something out of your comfort zone.

Feeling: Afraid, anxious, apprehensive, distressed, uncomfortable, worried.

WHAT HAPPENS TO THE BODY?

Inside: The amygdala, which is the part of the brain responsible for receiving incoming messages from your senses, detects threat or danger and sends a message to the hypothalamus. The hypothalamus is connected to the nervous system and triggers the fight-or-flight response. The enteric nervous system, which is the nerves connected to your stomach, is activated. The sympathetic nervous system, which releases stress hormones into the bloodstream and triggers fight or flight, is activated. The stress hormone cortisol, which pushes the body into action to combat stress, is released into the bloodstream. Adrenalin, which distributes blood away from the heart and to muscles in readiness for action, is released. The digestive, immune and reproductive systems slow down and are suppressed. Heart rate speeds up. Rapid breathing. Blood pressure rises. Blood vessels constrict. Muscles tense.

Outside: Body is restless.

Reaction: To be agitated.

Root Cause: Fear.

NUMB

Meaning: A mental and emotional process where you shut out your feelings so you cannot feel them anymore.

Purpose: To help you to separate the mind and body from any further hurt and pain.

Feeling: No emotion. (Emotional numbness can lead to dissociation, detachment and disconnection.)

What happens to the body?

Inside: The limbic system, which is the part of the brain that is responsible for processing emotions, deactivates. The amygdala, which is part of the limbic system and responsible for processing information from your senses for flight or flight, deactivates. The thalamus, which is the part of the brain responsible for feelings through temperature, touch, pain and pleasure, deactivates. The hippocampus, which is the part of the brain responsible for storing life experiences and how they feel in the body, deactivates. The circulatory system, which is responsible for the flow of blood and oxygen to the heart and brain, is disrupted. Heart rate slows. Breathing slows. Muscles tense.

Outside: Body is tense.

Reaction: To block (stop emotions flowing through you).

Root Cause: Fear.

OVERWHELMED

Meaning: A state of mind and being where you feel a wave of emotion that takes over you mentally, emotionally and physically.

Purpose: To help you be aware you are experiencing too many emotions at one time.

Feeling: Overpowered (extremely intense force washing over you).

What happens to the body?

Inside: The amygdala, which is the part of the brain responsible for receiving incoming messages from your senses, becomes overactivate. The nervous system is activated. The hypothalamus, which is the part of the brain connected to the nervous system and triggers the fight-or-flight response, is activated. The sympathetic nervous system, which is responsible for releasing hormones into the bloodstream, is activated. The stress hormone cortisol, which is responsible for pushing the body into action to combat stress, is released into the bloodstream. Adrenalin, which distributes blood away from the heart and to the muscles ready for action, is released. Noradrenaline, which mobilizes the brain and body for action in order to keep you safe, is released. The digestive, immune and reproductive systems slow down and are suppressed. Heart rate speeds up. Rapid breathing. Blood pressure rises. Blood vessels constrict. Muscles tense.

Outside: Body is restless.

Reaction: To freeze, fight or take flight.

Root Cause: Fear.

PANIC

Meaning: A state of mind and being where you feel a sudden and completely overpowering sensation that takes over your mind and makes your body move.

Purpose: To help you be aware that you are in danger and need to protect yourself.

Feeling: Anxiety, apprehensive, discomfort, frightened, scared, unsafe.

WHAT HAPPENS TO THE BODY?

Inside: The amygdala, which is the part of the brain responsible for receiving incoming messages, receives a warning of threat and danger and over-activates. It sends a message to the hypothalamus, which immediately triggers the fight-or-flight response. The frontal lobe part of the brain, which is responsible for personality, problem-solving and behaviour, is deactivated. The sympathetic nervous system, which prepares the body for fight and flight, is activated. Cortisol, which increases energy, is released into the bloodstream Adrenalin, which distributes blood to muscles is released. Noradrenaline, which is responsible for alertness and mobilizing the brain and body for action, is released. Heart rate speeds up. Rapid breathing. Blood pressure rises. Blood vessels constrict. Muscles tense. Peripheral vision is lost, causing tunnel vision. Hearing decreases.

Outside: Dizziness, shortness of breath, sweating, trembling.

Reaction: To fight or take flight.

Root Cause: Fear.

PETRIFIED

Meaning: A state of mind and being that gives you a feeling of being so frightened that you are unable to think or move.

Purpose: To help you be aware that you are experiencing something extremely scary.

Feeling: Terrified.

WHAT HAPPENS TO THE BODY?

Inside: The amygdala, which is the part of the brain responsible for receiving incoming messages from senses, receives a message of threat and danger and sends a message to the hypothalamus, which immediately triggers the fight-or-flight response. The frontal lobe of the brain, responsible for personality, thinking, problem-solving and behaviour, is immediately shut down. The pituitary gland, which releases stress hormones, becomes over activated. The sympathetic nervous system, which prepares the body for fight and flight, becomes over-activated. The stress hormone cortisol, which increases energy, is released into the bloodstream at full speed. The circulatory system, which is responsible for pushing blood through the body and pumping oxygen towards the heart

Dictionary

and brain, suddenly drops. Blood flow severely decreases; blood pressure severely decreases. The brain lacks blood flow and oxygen. The respiratory system, which is responsible for absorbing oxygen from air through the nose, mouth and lungs becomes over-activated. Heart rate drops. Rapid breathing. Muscles become very tense.

Outside: Body becomes numb and motionless.

Reaction: To freeze (become motionless or paralyzed).

Root Cause: Fear.

PITY

Meaning: A state of mind and being where you are sad for someone else's unhappiness, suffering or difficult situation. (There is also self-pity, where you feel sorry for yourself – blaming the outside world, rather than looking within.)

Purpose: To help you connect to another person's experience.

Feeling: Sorry.

WHAT HAPPENS TO THE BODY?

Inside: The cerebrum, which is the largest part of the brain and is responsible for thinking and feeling, as well as emotion and awareness, registers an awareness. The hippocampus, which is the part of the brain responsible for storing memory, is activated. The amygdala, which is the part of the brain responsible for emotions and behaviour, is activated. The hypothalamus, which is connected to your autonomic nervous system and regulates your breathing, heartbeat and digestion, is triggered. The parasympathetic nervous system, which slows the heart rate and increases gland activity, is activated. Heart rate slows. Breath decreases. Muscles contract.

Outside: Body lowers.

Reaction: To be sympathetic.
Root Cause: Sadness.

PRESSURED

Meaning: A state of mind and being that makes you feel as if someone or something is pushing on you mentally, emotionally and physically with a sense of urgency or high demand. (The pressures of life include family, peers, society, self and survival.)
Purpose: To help you to connect to your spirit.
Feeling: Stressed.

WHAT HAPPENS TO THE BODY?

Inside: The hypothalamus, which is the part of the brain responsible for emotional responses and releasing hormones into the bloodstream, is activated. The sympathetic nervous system, which stimulates the body's fight-or-flight response, is activated. The adrenal cortex, which releases the stress hormone cortisol into the bloodstream, is activated. Cortisol pushes the body into action to combat stress. Adrenalin, which distributes blood away from the heart and towards muscles in readiness for action, is released. Heart rate speeds up. Rapid breathing. Blood pressure rises. Blood vessels constrict. Muscles tense.
Outside: Body is pressured and weighed down.
Reaction: To break down or to push through.
Root Cause: Fear.

POWERLESS

Meaning: A state of mind and being where you feel you have no ability, no strength and no influence to act in an external situation or circumstance.
Purpose: To help you surrender to yourself; to help you find power from within.

Feeling: Helpless.

WHAT HAPPENS TO THE BODY?

Inside: The amygdala, which is the part of the brain responsible for receiving incoming messages from your senses and responds to fear, detects a threat and sends an immediate message to the hypothalamus. The hypothalamus, which is connected to your autonomic nervous system and unconsciously regulates your breathing, heartbeat and digestion, is triggered. The sympathetic nervous system, which stimulates the body's fight-or-flight response, is activated. Heart rate increases. Breathing speeds up, Blood pressure rises. Muscles contract. Blood vessels constrict.

Outside: Body is restless.

Reaction: To struggle, to fight or take flight.

Root Cause: Fear.

RAGE

Meaning: A state of mind and being where you feel you are facing a threatening situation.

Purpose: To give you the strength and power to make a change.

Feeling: Anger, fury. (Rage is an extreme expression of anger and can cause further pain and destruction.)

WHAT HAPPENS TO THE BODY?

Inside: The amygdala, which is the part of the brain responsible for receiving incoming messages from the senses, receives a message of a threat. The front lobe, which is the part of the brain responsible for personality, problem-solving and behaviour, is shut down. The hypothalamus, which is connected to your autonomic nervous system and unconsciously regulates your breathing, heartbeat and digestion, is triggered. The sympathetic nervous system, which stimulates the body's fight-or-flight response, is activated. The stress hormone cortisol – which is responsible for mood, motivation and emotions and alerting or shutting down body functions such as the digestive, immune and reproductive systems or growth processes – is released. The hormone adrenalin, which distributes blood to muscles in readiness for action, is released in high amounts. The hormone noradrenaline, which mobilizes the brain and body for action, is released. Heart rate increases. Breathing speeds up. Blood pressure rises. Muscles contract. Blood vessels constrict. Peripheral vision is lost, resulting in tunnel vision.

Outside: Pupils dilate, senses heighten, body is energized.

Reaction: To lash out.

Root Cause: Fear.

REGRET

Meaning: An emotional state of mind and being that makes you feel bad about something you have done or said.

Purpose: To help you be aware of your actions and of the consequences.

Feeling: Disappointed, guilty.

WHAT HAPPENS TO THE BODY?

Inside: The cerebrum – which is the largest part of the brain and responsible for thinking and feeling, as well as emotion and awareness – registers an awareness that something does not feel right. The hippocampus, which is the part of the brain responsible for storing memory, is activated. The amygdala, which is the part of the brain responsible for emotions and behaviour, is activated. The hypothalamus, which is the part of your brain connected to your autonomic nervous system that regulates your breathing, heartbeat and digestion, is triggered. The parasympathetic nervous system, which slows your heart rate and increases gland activity, is activated. Heart rate slows. Breathing slows. Muscles contract.

Outside: Body slumps.

Reaction: To repent (feel sorry for any wrongdoing).

Root Cause: Sadness.

REMORSE

Meaning: A state of mind and being where you feel bad for something that has happened or something you have said or done

Purpose: To make you aware of actions, reactions and their consequences.

Feeling: Shame, unhappy, regret.

WHAT HAPPENS TO THE BODY?

Inside: The cerebrum, which is the largest part of the brain and responsible for thinking and feeling, as well as emotion and awareness, registers an awareness that something does not feel right. The hippocampus, which is the part of the brain responsible for storing memory, is activated. The amygdala, which is the part of the brain responsible for emotions and behaviour, is activated. The hypothalamus, which is the part of your brain connected to your autonomic nervous system that regulates your breathing, heartbeat and digestion, is triggered. The parasympathetic nervous system, which slows your heart rate and increases gland activity, is activated. Heart rate slows. Breathing slows. Muscles contract.

Outside: Body slumps.

Reaction: To apologize.

Root Cause: Sadness.

Resentment

Meaning: A state of being where you are aware you are holding on to a bad experience.

Purpose: To help you be aware that you did not like what you experienced.

Feeling: Angry, bitter, hurt, hatred, powerless. (Resentment can carry many emotions like anger, sadness, hurt and pain, and this can have a huge impact and influence on your mind and body; it is important for you to find a way to release resentment.)

What happens to the body?

Inside: The hippocampus, which is the part of the brain responsible for repeating episodic memories, is activated. The amygdala, which is responsible for processing emotions, becomes overactivate. The thalamus, which is responsible for triggering emotions related to past events, is activated. The somatosensory cortex, which is the part of the brain that receives and processes sensory information from the entire body, is activated. The endocrine system, which releases hormones into the bloodstream and works in balance with the immune system and the nervous system, is disrupted. The cardiovascular system, which pumps blood to the heart and brain, slows down. The respiratory system, which helps you breathe, slows down. Heart rate slows. Breathing slows. Muscles constrict. Blood flow is restricted.

Outside: Body is tense.

Reaction: To resent.

Root Cause: Fear, sadness.

Dictionary

SENSITIVE

Meaning: An emotional state of mind and being where you feel deeply and instantly detect or respond to the slightest change.

Purpose: To help you to heighten your awareness.

Feeling: Overwhelmed.

WHAT HAPPENS TO THE BODY?

Inside: The amygdala, which is the part of the brain responsible for receiving incoming messages from your senses, becomes overactivate. The nervous system is activated. The hypothalamus, which is the part of the brain connected to the nervous system and which triggers fight or flight, is activated. The sympathetic nervous system, which releases hormones into the bloodstream, is activated. The stress hormone cortisol, which pushes the body into action to combat stress, is released into the bloodstream. The hormone adrenalin, which distributes the blood away from the heart and toward the muscles in readiness for action, is released. Noradrenaline, which mobilizes the brain and body for action and to keep you safe, is released. The digestive, immune and reproductive systems slow down and are suppressed. Heart rate increases. Rapid breathing. Blood pressure rises. Blood vessels constrict. Muscles tense.

Outside: Body is sensitive.

Reaction: To absorb, to fight or take flight.

Root Cause: Fear.

SHAME

Meaning: A state of mind and being that makes you feel exposed for doing something wrong.

Purpose: To help you be aware of yourself and your actions and reactions.

Feeling: Embarrassed, guilty, foolish.

WHAT HAPPENS TO THE BODY?

Inside: The amygdala, which is the part of the brain responsible for processing emotions and behaviour, is activated. The hypothalamus, which is responsible for triggering the fight-or-flight response, is activated. The insula, which is the part of the brain responsible for perception and pain, is activated. The hippocampus, which is the part of the brain responsible for storing memories, is activated. The sympathetic nervous system, which releases hormones into the bloodstream and activates the fight-or-flight response, is activated. The stress hormone cortisol, which pushes the body into action to combat stress, is released into the bloodstream. Heart rate increases. Rapid breathing. Blood pressure rises. Blood vessels constrict. Muscles tense. Peripheral vision is lost, causing tunnel vision. Hearing decreases.

Outside: Body tenses.

Reaction: To be ashamed, to fight or take flight.

Root cause: Fear.

SHOCK

Meaning: A state of mind and being where you experience something that is sudden and unexpected and it is too much for the mind and body to handle.

Purpose: To help you to protect yourself in unexpected and difficult experiences.

Feeling: Numb, overwhelmed.

Dictionary

WHAT HAPPENS TO THE BODY?
Inside: The circulatory system, which is responsible for ensuring blood flows through the body and oxygen is pumped toward the heart and brain, suddenly slows down. Blood flow is severely decreased. Blood pressure severely decreases. Brain lacks blood flow and oxygen. The respiratory system, which is responsible for absorbing oxygen through the nose, mouth and lungs, becomes over-activated. Heart rate drops. Breathing speeds up. Muscles become very tense.
Outside: Body freezes (becomes motionless or paralyzed).
Reaction: To go numb.
Root Cause: Fear, sadness.

SHY
Meaning: A state of mind and being where you feel extremely uncomfortable in a situation.
Purpose: To help you to step inside of your whole self and find your power.
Feeling: Nervous, insecure.
WHAT HAPPENS TO THE BODY?
Inside: The amygdala, which is the part of the brain responsible for responding to fear, is immediately activated. The sympathetic nervous system, which prepares the body for fight or flight, is activated. The stress hormone cortisol, which helps the body respond to stress, is activated and released into the bloodstream. Heartbeat quickens. Rapid breathing. Blood vessels dilate with increased blood flow towards skin.
Outside: Face blushes, breathless, body is shaky, speechless.
Reaction: To withdraw.
Root Cause: Fear.

Sorrow

Meaning: A state of mind and being where you are feeling a deep sadness caused by some form of loss, or a feeling of misfortune or suffering.

Purpose: To help you be aware of a loss and the movement of life and change.

Feeling: Anguish, unhappy, depressed.

What happens to the body?

Inside: The hippocampus, which is part of the brain responsible for storing your life stories, memories and associations, is activated. The amygdala, which is the part of the brain responsible for fear and triggering the fight-or-flight response, becomes over activated. The nervous system, which keeps your body in a homeostasis state and balances the body system, becomes disrupted. The sympathetic nervous system, which releases the stress hormones cortisol and adrenalin into your bloodstream, is disrupted. The parasympathetic nervous system, which is responsible for conserving energy in your body and the body's rest and digestion response, is underactive or overactive. The circulatory system, which circulates blood to your heart and brain and throughout your body, is disrupted. The immune and digestive systems are disrupted. Heart rate is Irregular. Breathing is irregular. Blood pressure rises, muscles tense.

Outside: Body is restless.

Reaction: To be distressed.

Root Cause: Sadness.

Stressed

Meaning: A state of mind and being where you are experiencing a mental, emotional, or physical strain. (Acute stress is short term; chronic stress is long term.)

Dictionary

Purpose: To help you move forward; to help you adapt and make decisions. (If you stay in a state of stress for a long period of time it will impact on your physical body.)

Feeling: Nervous, worried.

WHAT HAPPENS TO THE BODY?

Inside: The hypothalamic-pituitary-adrenal (HPA) axis, which is the central stress response system that interconnects the brain, the nervous system and the endocrine system, is immediately activated. The hypothalamus, which is part of the brain responsible for emotional responses and releasing hormones into the bloodstream (and is part of the HPA Axis circuit), is activated. The anterior pituitary gland, which is responsible for releasing stress hormones into the bloodstream, is activated. The adrenal cortex, which is responsible for releasing the stress hormone cortisol into the bloodstream, is activated; cortisol pushes the body into action to combat stress. The hormone adrenalin, which distributes blood away from the heart and towards muscles in readiness for action, is released. The digestive, immune and reproductive systems are suppressed. Heart rate speeds up. Rapid breathing. Blood pressure rises. Blood vessels constrict. Muscles tense.

Outside: Headaches, upset stomach, chest pain, insomnia, loss of sexual desire.

Reaction: To be restless, weighed down, burdened.

Root Cause: Fear.

TERRIFIED

Meaning: A state of mind and being where you are extremely scared.

Purpose: To help you be aware of a threat or danger.

Feeling: Afraid, panicked.

WHAT HAPPENS TO THE BODY?

Inside: The amygdala, which is the part of the brain responsible for receiving incoming messages, receives a message of threat and danger and sends a message to the hypothalamus, which immediately triggers the fight-or-flight response. The pituitary gland, which releases the stress hormones cortisol and adrenalin, is activated. The sympathetic nervous system, which prepares the body for fight or flight, is activated. The immune, digestive and reproductive systems are suppressed. Heart rate speeds up. Rapid breathing. Blood pressure rises. Blood vessels constrict. Muscles tense. Peripheral vision is lost, causing tunnel vision. Hearing decreases.

Outside: Body trembles and shakes.

Reaction: To freeze, to fight or take flight.

Root Cause: Fear.

THREATENED

Meaning: A state of mind and being where you feel as if someone is trying to cause you harm.

Purpose: To help protect you from uncomfortable, risky or dangerous situations.

Feeling: Angry, anxious, vulnerable.

WHAT HAPPENS TO THE BODY?

Inside: The amygdala, which is the part of the brain responsible for receiving incoming messages, receives a message of threat and danger and sends a message to the hypothalamus, which immediately triggers the fight-or-flight response. The pituitary gland, which releases the stress hormones cortisol and adrenalin, is activated. The sympathetic nervous system, which prepares the body for fight or flight, is activated. The immune, digestive and reproductive systems are suppressed. Heart rate speeds up. Rapid breathing. Blood pressure rises. Blood vessels constrict. Muscles tense. Peripheral vision is lost, causing tunnel vision. Hearing decreases.

Outside: Body is on high alert ready for action.

Reaction: To defend, to protect.

Root Cause: Fear.

Torn

Meaning: A state of mind and being where you are being pulled in different directions.

Purpose: To help you to surrender and go within and connect to your core.

Feeling: Conflicted.

What happens to the body?

Inside: The prefrontal cortex, which is the part of the brain responsible for attention and focus, fires messages back and forth to the amygdala. The amygdala sends continuous messages of potential threat to the hypothalamus. The hypothalamus, which is the part of the brain responsible for releasing hormones and actioning the flight-or-fight response, sends a message to the body to prepare for a threat. The autonomic nervous system, which regulates your heart, breathing, digestion and pupil responses, activates your sympathetic nervous system, which triggers the fight-or-flight response. The stress hormones cortisol and adrenalin are released into the bloodstream. Blood vessels constrict. Muscles tense. Heartbeat is irregular. Breathing is irregular.

Outside: Body is restless, head is unclear and can ache.

Root Cause: Fear.

TROUBLED

Meaning: A state of mind and being where you feel you are in a situation that is causing you difficulty.

Purpose: To help you be aware that you need to find a solution.

Feeling: Anxious, confused, distressed, disturbed, upset, worried.

WHAT HAPPENS TO THE BODY?

Inside: The amygdala, which is the part of the brain responsible for receiving incoming messages from your senses, detects threat and sends a message to the hypothalamus. The hypothalamus is connected to the nervous system and the fight-or-flight response is activated. The sympathetic nervous system, which is responsible for releasing hormones into the bloodstream is activated. The stress hormone cortisol, which pushes the body into action to combat stress, is released into the bloodstream. The hormone adrenalin, which distributes blood away from the heart and towards the muscles in readiness for action, is released. The digestive, immune and reproductive systems are suppressed. Heart rate speeds up. Rapid breathing. Blood pressure rises. Blood vessels constrict. Muscles tense.

Outside: Body is restless.

Reaction: To worry.

Root Cause: Fear.

TRAPPED

Meaning: A state of mind and being where you feel you are in an unpleasant situation that lacks freedom, and you cannot move or escape from it.

Purpose: To help you be aware that you are feeling restricted (limited in what you can do and/or where you can go).

Feeling: Anxious, hopeless, powerless.

What happens to the body?

Inside: The amygdala, which is the part of the brain responsible for receiving incoming messages from your senses, detects threat and sends a message to the hypothalamus. The hypothalamus is connected to the nervous system and the fight-or-flight response is activated. The sympathetic nervous system, which is responsible for releasing hormones into the bloodstream, is activated. The stress hormone cortisol, which pushes the body into action to combat stress, is released into the bloodstream. The hormone adrenalin, which distributes blood away from the heart and toward the muscles in readiness for action is released. The digestive, immune and reproductive systems are suppressed. Heart rate speeds up. Rapid breathing. Blood pressure rises. Blood vessels constrict. Muscles tense.

Outside: Body is restless.

Reaction: To fight or take flight.

Root Cause: Fear.

TRAUMATIZED

Meaning: A state of mind and being where you are suffering from the aftermath of a bad, unpleasant, painful experience. (If trauma is not processed, it can trap itself in the mind and body, causing them to experience shock, distress, discomfort and pain. If this trauma is not in your awareness or remains unhealed, as time passes your mind and body will continue to be impacted by this trauma. Your emotions, thoughts, and memories attached to the trauma can start playing back to you or revealing themselves to you in some way.)

Purpose: To help you be aware that you have not processed or are not processing what you have experienced.

Feeling: Angry, anguish, shocked, hurt.

WHAT HAPPENS TO THE BODY?

Inside: The amygdala, which is the part of the brain that is responsible for receiving incoming messages, receives a message of threat and danger. The front lobe, which is the part of the brain responsible for personality, problem-solving and behaviour, is deactivated. The nervous system, which regulates the fight-or-flight response and releasing hormones into the bloodstream and maintains balance in the body, is disrupted. The sympathetic nervous system, which prepares the body for fight or flight, is activated. The endocrine system, which releases hormones into the bloodstream to balance the body, is disrupted. The stress hormone cortisol, which increases energy in the bloodstream is released. Adrenalin, which distributes blood to the muscles, is released. Noradrenaline, which is responsible for alertness and mobilizing the brain and body for action, is released. The immune, digestive and reproductive systems are suppressed. Heart rate speeds up. Rapid breathing. Blood pressure rises. Blood vessels constrict. Muscles tense. Peripheral vision is lost, causing tunnel vision. Hearing decreases.

Outside: Body is on high alert, body is hyper-aroused, body is restless.

Reaction: To be traumatized.

Root Cause: Fear, sadness.

UNEASY

Meaning: A state of mind and being where you are feeling discomfort.

Purpose: To make you aware you are not in a comfortable, familiar place.

Dictionary

Feeling: Agitated, anxious, disturbed, troubled.

WHAT HAPPENS TO THE BODY?

Inside: The amygdala, which is the part of the brain responsible for receiving incoming messages from your senses, detects threat and sends a message to the hypothalamus. The hypothalamus is connected to the nervous system, and the fight-or-flight response is activated. The sympathetic nervous system, which is responsible for releasing hormones into the bloodstream, is activated. The stress hormone cortisol, which pushes the body into action to combat stress, is released into the bloodstream. The hormone adrenalin, which distributes blood away from the heart and towards the muscles in readiness for action, is released. The digestive, immune and reproductive systems are suppressed. Heart rate speeds up. Rapid breathing. Blood pressure rises. Blood vessels constrict. Muscles tense.

Outside: Body is tense.

Reaction: To be on guard (watching over to control or protect).

Root cause: Fear.

UNFULFILLED

Meaning: A state of mind and being where you feel you are incomplete.

Purpose: To help you be aware that there is something missing in your life.

Feeling: Empty, unhappy.

WHAT HAPPENS TO THE BODY?

Inside: The amygdala, which is the part of the brain responsible for processing emotion and behaviour and assessing the environment, detects unhappiness and alerts the hippocampus. The hippocampus, which is the part of the brain responsible for storing episodic memories, triggers a past experience to help your body to respond to a similar situation. The parasympathetic nervous system, which slows heart rate and increases gland activity, is activated. Heartbeat slows. Breathing slows. Blood vessels constrict. Blood pressure rises. Muscles tense. Blood flow decreases.

Outside: Body slumps.

Reaction: To search.

Root cause: Sadness.

UNHAPPY

Meaning: A state of mind and being that makes you feel you are not happy.

Purpose: To help you be aware that you are not where you want to be in life.

Feeling: Discontent, dissatisfied, unfulfilled.

WHAT HAPPENS TO THE BODY?

Inside: The amygdala, which is the part of the brain responsible for processing emotion and behaviour and assessing the environment, detects unhappiness and alerts the hippocampus. The hippocampus, which is the part of the brain responsible for storing life memories, triggers a past experience to help your body respond to a similar situation. The parasympathetic nervous system, which slows the heart rate and increases gland activity, is activated. Heartbeat slows. Breathing slows. Blood vessels constrict. Blood pressure rises. Muscles tense. Blood flow decreases.

Outside: Body slumps.

Reaction: To withdraw.

Root cause: Sadness.

Dictionary

UNLOVED

Meaning: A strong feeling that makes you feel you are not cared for or loved.

Purpose: To help you to find a way to love and care for yourself and to connect to your whole self. (A chronic feeling of being unloved can lead you into deeper layers of negative states and deeper into situations where you will feel a need to defend and protect yourself. This can lead to aggressive behaviour and words that do not align with who you are, and that is not who you are at the core.)

Feeling: Isolated, lonely, unhappy.

WHAT HAPPENS TO THE BODY?

Inside: The amygdala, which is the part of the brain responsible for processing emotion and behaviour and assessing the environment, detects a feeling of no love and alerts the hippocampus. The hippocampus, which is the part of the brain responsible for storing life memories, triggers a past experience to help your body respond to a similar situation. The sympathetic nervous system, which prepares the body for fight or flight, is triggered. The endocrine system, which releases hormones into the bloodstream and works in balance with the immune system and nervous system is disrupted. The stress hormones cortisol and adrenalin are released into the bloodstream. The cardiovascular system, which pumps blood to the heart and brain, is disrupted. The respiratory system, which helps you breathe, is disrupted. Heart rate and breathing are irregular. Muscles constrict. Blood flow is restricted.

Outside: Body is on guard, body is tense.

Reaction: To defend, to protect.

Root Cause: Fear, sadness.

UNSAFE

Meaning: A state of mind and being that makes you feel that you are in harm or danger.

Purpose: To help you to be aware that you do not feel safe.

Feeling: Frightened, insecure, scared, vulnerable.

WHAT HAPPENS TO THE BODY?

Inside: The amygdala, which is the part of the brain responsible for receiving incoming messages, receives a message of threat and danger. The sympathetic nervous system, which prepares the body for fight or flight, is activated. The pituitary gland, which releases stress hormones, is activated. The stress hormone cortisol, which pushes the body into action to combat stress, is released into the bloodstream. The hormone adrenalin, which distributes blood away from the heart and towards muscles in readiness for action, is released. The hormone noradrenaline, which mobilizes the brain and body for action in order to keep you safe, is released. The immune, digestive and reproductive systems are suppressed. Heart rate speeds up. Rapid breathing. Blood pressure rises. Blood vessels constrict. Muscles tense.

Outside: Body is on high alert.

Reaction: To defend, to protect.

Root cause: Fear.

VULNERABLE

Meaning: A mental state of mind and being where you feel you are exposed, laid out bare, to attack or harm.

Purpose: To help you be aware that you are in a place or position that leaves you open to injury, damage or hurt.

Feeling: Unsafe.

What happens to the body?

Inside: The amygdala, which is the part of the brain responsible for receiving incoming messages, receives a message of threat and danger. The sympathetic nervous system, which prepares the body for fight or flight, is activated. The pituitary gland, which releases stress hormones, is activated. The stress hormone cortisol, which pushes the body into action to combat stress, is released into the bloodstream. The hormone adrenalin, which distributes blood away from the heart and toward muscles in readiness for action, is released. The hormone noradrenaline, which mobilizes the brain and body for action in order to keep you safe, is released. The immune, digestive and reproductive systems are suppressed. Heart rate speeds up. Rapid breathing. Blood pressure rises. Blood vessels constrict. Muscles tense.

Outside: Body is restless.

Reaction: To protect.

Root Cause: Fear.

Worried

Meaning: A state of mind and being where you keep thinking about problems or unpleasant things.

Purpose: To help you be aware that there is a problem in your life that needs solving.

Feeling: Anxious, stressed, troubled.

What happens to the body?

Inside: The amygdala, which is the part of the brain responsible for receiving incoming messages from your senses, detects worry and sends a message to the hypothalamus. The hypothalamus is connected to the nervous system, and the fight-or-flight response is activated. The sympathetic nervous system, which releases hormones into the bloodstream, is activated. The stress hormone cortisol, which pushes the body into action to combat stress, is released into the bloodstream. The hormone adrenalin, which distributes blood away from the heart and toward muscles in readiness for action, is released. The immune, digestive and reproductive systems are suppressed. Heart rate speeds up. Rapid breathing. Blood pressure rises. Blood vessels constrict. Muscles tense.

Outside: Forehead muscles tighten, pupils constrict, body tenses.
Reaction: To be restless.
Root Cause: Fear.

Negative reactions and responses

When you feel bad inside your mind and body, you may experience some of the following reactions and responses. If you are unaware of how you feel, and cannot pinpoint it, or find a name, see your reaction, this can help you to understand how you really, feel and what is happening.

REACTION	RESPONSE
Attack	act against
Begrudge	give reluctantly or resentfully
Agitated	be troubled
Beaten	be worn down
Belittle	dismiss (someone or something) as unimportant
Blame	feel that someone or something is responsible and is at fault or wrong
Cautious	be careful
Crumble	break or fall apart

Dictionary

Crumple	crease and wrinkle, or to fall
Demoralized	lose confidence or hope
Demotivated	be less eager
Disorientated	lose your sense of direction
Distracted	take your attention away to someplace else
Distressed	suffer from an emotional pain
Distrust	feel that someone or something cannot be relied upon
Fight	take part in a violent struggle
Flight	flee
Freeze	be motionless
Fury	feel extreme anger
Grudge	persistently feel ill will or resentment due to a past experience
Hide	be out of sight
High Alert	be on guard, watchful
Inadequate	unable to deal with a situation or with life
Lacking	be in short supply
Lash out	attack with words or action
Lose Faith	lose complete trust or confidence in someone or something
Lower Mood	move in a downward direction
Overwhelmed	experience a strong emotional effect
Pessimistic	see the worst aspect of things or believe the worst will happen
Reject	dismiss or push away
Resent	be bitter
Resist	exert force in opposition
Restless	unable to rest or relax
Self-Conscious	feel undue awareness of oneself, one's appearance, or one's actions
Spite	wish to hurt, annoy or offend someone
Strongly react	respond to something with an emotion that is too strong or an action that is unnecessary
Tense	feel tight and rigid
Traumatized	feel persistent negative emotions as a result of disturbing experiences
Uncertain	be unsure
Unclear	not easy to see, hear or understand

Unsettled	lack order and stability
Upset	be unhappy
Uptight	feel tense and overly controlled
Vindictive	desire revenge
Violated	break or act against something
Withdraw	remove yourself from a particular place or thing
Yearn	long for something, typically something that one has lost or been separated from

If you feel bad in mind and body, it is natural for you to want to:

- attack
- begrudge
- blame
- distrust
- fight or take flight
- lash out
- lose faith
- reject
- tense

A final note on negative

Negative emotions and feelings can feel painful and uncomfortable, and can feel heavy, especially as they layer over each other. When this happens, it can feel as if life is hard and not going your way. This is not true. Your emotional states are here to guide you and help you in life; to protect you from danger; and to drive you in new ways, and help you find new ways of seeing – to help you develop, grow and evolve. If you keep this in mind when you start to feel bad in mind and body, you can start to experience your negative emotions and feelings differently. Working with them can help you find a way to move through the negative state. Do not get lost or stuck with them, rather work your way through the layers of negative states and come out the other end to see your power, your strength, and all that you are mentally, emotionally, physically and spiritually.

THE BLANK CANVAS: NEGATIVE

Each time you find yourself visiting the Negative dictionary because you have experienced one of the emotions or feelings above, and you have sat with the emotion or feeling, then take a moment to place the name of the feeling (or even just a tick) in the circle to remind yourself of that feeling.

Negative:

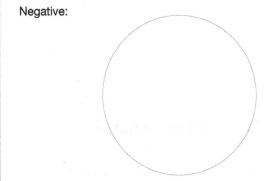

CHAPTER 7
HOW DO YOU FEEL AS A WHOLE?

THE BLANK CANVAS:
DICTIONARY OF FEELINGS

Use the empty space below to note down what this chapter has made you think about and how it has made you feel.

Did you experience any emotions or feelings?

Did you form any new or surprising thoughts or opinions?

Did you come to any conclusions or judgements?

Use the space below to expose, truthfully and clearly, your internal narrative – make it seen.

THE BLANK CANVAS: POSITIVE, NEUTRAL AND NEGATIVE

Now, go back to the positive, neutral and negative circles that I asked you to make a note or a tick in each time you felt an emotion or feeling. Count the emotions/ticks. If you did not fill out these parts, please take the time to do so, and you will see your emotional self.

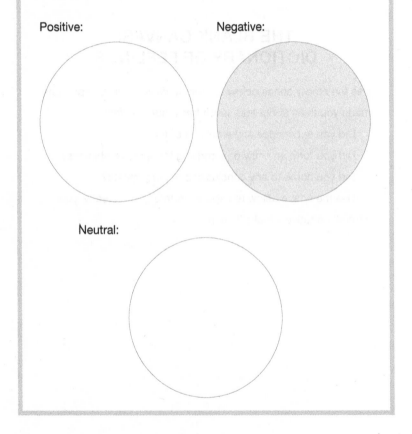

Positive:

Negative:

Neutral:

All the words you have read in Part 1 will help you understand Part 2.

PART 2

HOW TO WORK SUCCESSFULLY WITH YOUR WHOLE SELF (BEING PRACTICAL)

Part 2 will help you to work successfully with your mental, emotional, physical, spiritual and whole self.

To "work" means to engage in a mental, emotional, physical and/or spiritual activity.

To "work with" means to engage in that activity together or in the same direction as.

To "work successfully with" means to engage in in a way that helps achieve positive results.

Part 2 will also help you with:

- **Observation**: looking carefully at what is happening to you
- **Introspection**: analysing and examining your whole self
- **Exercises**: engaging in activities or tasks to make a positive change
- **Practices**: engaging in new ways of trying things and repeating them so they become your way
- **Checking in**: turning inwards and checking in with yourself mentally, emotionally, physically and spiritually

What you need to know about Part 2

BOXES

There will be many phrases in boxes. You might wonder why. This has purpose and meaning: in a world where there is information overload and a lot to process, framing particular words will make it easier for our minds to remember and digest them. Creating a visual effect will help you to bring these words to the front of your mind, and to remember what you need to see or change or work with. It is a simple, but effective way of helping you to work with yourself.

EXERCISES

There are short exercises to help you take short, practical steps to _start_ working successfully with your whole self.

NB: If you are seeking a guide to help you with some deeper issues and deeper layers of healing, or deep trauma and deeper layers of inner work, I recommend you seek professional help. You can also use this part of the guide alongside professional help.

8

HOW TO SUCCESSFULLY START WORKING WITH YOUR WHOLE SELF

Step 4: Learn how to work "with" and not "against" yourself.

Awaken

Awaken means to:

- wake up from sleep
- become aware of
- come into existence

WHAT DOES IT MEAN TO AWAKEN?

It means to awaken to how you think, react, act and behave as a whole, in all of your:

- mind
- body
- spirit

- instincts
- senses
- emotions
- feelings
- thoughts
- behaviours

It means to awaken to your whole self – to see clearly what is happening so you do not keep reacting from an unconscious or autopilot state.

This means waking up to any reactions, actions, habits, patterns and behaviours that do not align with your truth or align with your true nature. It is to wake up and see beyond the surface of how you portray yourself, and dig deep through the layers of conditioning that have been passed down to you that you keep using but no longer help you or serve you, or keep you stuck or in pain.

HOW TO AWAKEN – OBSERVATION

Observation means the mental process of closely observing or monitoring what is happening without forming any words, criticism, judgement or without creating reaction.

Observing means to:

- look carefully, pay attention
- make no judgements
- have a neutral, open mind
- make no reaction, action or input

EXERCISE 1: OBSERVE YOUR THOUGHTS

As you wake up from sleep and open your eyes, start the observation process.

- *What words enter my mind?*
- *What is the natural flow of words to my mind – the streamline?*
- *What is the thought narrative in my mind?*
- *What is the story that is unfolding in my mind as I wake up?*

As you move through your day, keep observing the thoughts that enter your mind.

Ask yourself:

- *What is happening inside of my mind?*
- *What am I thinking in my mind?*
- *Is there a cycle or loop – thoughts that go round in a circle and come back to the same starting point?*
- *Is there a pattern (repeating thoughts)?*

EXERCISE 2: OBSERVE YOUR EMOTIONS AND FEELINGS

As you experience each thought, explore the layer beneath:

- *What are emotions and feelings attached to your thoughts?*
- *To what emotion or feeling do your thoughts lead you to?*

If you cannot go straight to exploring this layer, start with asking:

- *Does your mind feel good, neutral or bad?*

If your mind feels good, your thoughts are, or are leading toward, a positive state.

If your mind is neutral, then your thoughts have no emotion yet, but can lead toward a negative or positive state.

If your mind feels bad, your thoughts are in or are leading toward a negative state.

Start to observe the emotions and feelings that lie underneath your words.

Start to observe the emotions and feelings that are stirring in your mind and body.

As you move through your day, keep observing your emotions and feelings, the ones beneath the words or the ones that stir in your mind and body as life is happening to you both inside and out. Just observe – no other reaction or action is needed.

EXERCISE 3: OBSERVE YOUR REACTIONS AND ACTIONS

As you start the process of observing your thoughts and words, and as you experience the energy and sensations of your emotions and feelings, observe how your mind and body move and react and act, inside and out.

Notice how emotions, feelings and thoughts place your mind and body in a reactive mode.

EXERCISE 4: OBSERVE YOUR WHOLE SELF

Start to observe your whole self as if you are watching yourself from above, and observe:

- Your mind
- Your body

- Your spirit
- How do you feel?
- Your emotions and feelings
- Your thoughts
- Your reactions, actions and behaviours
- Your instincts and senses
- Yourself on the inside
- Yourself on the outside

Be AWARE

How do I feel?
Emotions
Feelings

How do I think?
Thoughts
Opinions
Judgments
Beliefs

How do I speak?
Words
Languages

How do I react?
Triggers
Alerts
Pain

> How do I behave?
>
> Outer persona
>
> Character
>
> Habits

When the day is over, just before you sleep, take some quiet time to reflect on the beginning of the day and how the day unfolded. What did you see? What was new to you that you had not seen before?

Ask yourself five questions:

1 **How do I think?** *What are my thoughts, judgements, opinions, beliefs?*
2 **How do I feel?** *What are my feelings, sensations, triggers, vibrations?*
3 **How do I speak?** *What words did I form and speak today?*
4 **How do I react?** *Are there triggers, alerts, alarms or pain?*
5 **How do I behave?** *How am I acting outwardly? What character am I being? What habits am I showing?*

The very next day, I advise you to wake up and start the whole process again. Try to do this exercise for a minimum of 30 days so you can start to observe how you think, move, speak, react, act, behave and connect.

After 30 days, you should start to see parts of yourself that you did not previously see or pay attention to – these take time to reveal themselves.

As you slowly start to awaken to yourself, you will start to see:

- all the parts of you that you are working with
- all the parts of you that you are working against
- which parts are in alignment with you as a whole

- which parts are in misalignment with you as a whole
- which parts of you are struggling to evolve and change
- which parts of you are untrue and not you, a lie
- which parts of you are hidden and are hurting, in pain
- which parts of you are being blocked and stuck inside
- which parts of you need help to be seen and understood
- which parts of you are not revealed – the unspoken, the unsaid

Each day will be different. The day will unfold in many ways – sometimes unexpected ways, new ways or repeated ways. You will start to notice what is happening to you; you will start to pay attention to how you react and act and behave. You will start to see where you are struggling or hurting. You will start to see when your mind and body move into a negative state and feel bad and are in pain and then react in an unconscious way.

This 30-day observation exercise will help you to awaken to your whole self. It will help you to be:

Conscious: aware of yourself and your surroundings, and of yourself and others

Aware: see and know and understand what is happening to you inside and out,

Self-Aware: understand yourself as a whole – your emotions, feelings, thoughts, reactions, behaviours

The exercise will also help you to understand why it is so important to learn to see your whole self clearly, and will help you to see how observation will help you work successfully with your mental, emotional, physical, spiritual and energetic self.

Journal

It is important you keep a journal of what you experience so you can reflect back on yourself when doing other exercises and practices to help you move forward.

CREATE A SPACE IN BETWEEN

What is "a space in between"?

As you experience life and react and act in response to what is happening to you, instead of reacting and acting in your usual way or in an automatic or unconscious way, you pause and create a space between what is happening and your response to it.

It is in this space of the pause that you can take a moment to ask yourself:

- *Is this who I am?*
- *Am I being me?*
- *Is this who I want to be?*

In this space you create for yourself you gain:

A CHANCE. A CHOICE. A CHANGE.

a **Chance** – another way for something to happen

a **Choice** – the opportunity to choose which way you want to be or go.

a **Change** – the opportunity to react in a different way

9
HOW TO SUCCESSFULLY WORK WITH YOUR MENTAL SELF

Step 4: Learn how to work "with" and not "against" your mind.

Mental – your mind

Your mind is an extremely powerful force that is connected to another unseen powerful force that lies beyond this physical world. Your mind is intertwined with and connected to your body, your spirit, your senses, your emotions, your feelings, your reactions and actions and your behaviour. Your mind is connected to life. Your mind has experienced and seen and perceived and felt and been through a lot in your life.

Your mind:
   observes: sees all that is happening in your life: past, present, future.
   perceives: understands the world its own way, based on your senses and point of view.
   thinks: has thoughts and ideas and forms words, beliefs, opinions, conclusions and judgements.

feels: connects your experiences to your feelings.

stores: collects your life experiences, movements, memories, learnings, beliefs, skills, habits and patterns.

Your mind is:

conscious: aware and responding to your environment and surroundings.

subconscious: storing your life experiences, movements, memories, teachings, beliefs, skills, habits, patterns, reactions, actions, behaviours and learnings.

unconscious: unaware of what is happening, yet automatically responds.

Your mind has been influenced and impacted by:

emotions: mental states that feel good, neutral or bad

thoughts: a creation of words in your mind

experiences: events, circumstances, situations, outcomes

perception: the way you understand something through your senses

perspective: the way you view something from your position

senses: the way you see, hear, smell, touch, taste

thoughts: movement of mind in thoughts and ideas

life views: the ability to see something from a particular place

life position: a place where you are and where you stand

and further by:

beliefs: an acceptance of how something is– its truth

conclusions: decisions reached

opinions: personal views formed in the mind

judgements: final conclusions on how something is

narrative: a mental story that is created in your mind
teachings: ideas, knowledge, facts taught to you by others

Your mind is always seeking:

meaning
understanding
connection
familiarity
safety
security

The mental struggle

When you are engaged in a mental struggle, you struggle to find meaning or understanding in your experiences.

You struggle with what you are **perceiving**, it does not make sense to you.

You struggle to understand your **emotions** and the state of mind you are in.

You cannot **think** clearly – you find it hard to connect your mind to your reality. Your thoughts cloud your mind and take up mental space. Your thoughts are:

abnormal
unhealthy
unrealistic
distracted
intrusive
negative
repetitive

You feel **unsafe** – your mind is on high alert, ready to protect and disconnect.

You get **stuck in patterns** – the way you think, your thoughts, ideas, experiences.

You **spiral** into a low mood, and you fall into layers of negative emotions.

You are suffering as you struggle to overcome, hardship, hurt, loss, pain or unpleasant experiences.

MINDSET

Mindset can be:

open: allows room for more thoughts in your mind.

narrow: limited in the amount of thoughts your mind will allow.

growing: your mind is in the process of increasing the amount of thoughts it allows.

fixed: your thoughts are secured in position in your mind and unable to move.

closed: your mind is shut off to new thoughts.

Your mind can be:

blocked: thoughts are congested, making it difficult to work with them to create flow.

stuck: thoughts are hard to move from their fixed positions.

evolving: thoughts are moving and developing gradually.

A sacred space

Your mind is a sacred space; you should try to keep it clear and clean and pure. This is essential for your mental health and wellbeing and, more importantly, it is essential for your connection to your body and spirit.

Why do I say this?

An overload of information fed into the mind does not give your mind the space it needs to naturally connect to the body and spirit; it can also block the connection to your intuition, which is your inner voice that connects you to your whole self and helps you to go within to find your answers in life. If your attention is used to seeking outside information to help you make sense of what is happening, your mind will keep seeking answers on the outside of yourself, and this will imbalance the mind-body-spirit connection. You will not connect to your whole self.

To stay true to yourself, and balanced in life, you need to stay aligned with your whole self, not just your mind. If your mind is conditioned or is in an emotional state, this can influence your choices and decisions in life. It is also important to always remember and understand that your mind is not always influenced in the present moment, as the past can creep into your present and start influencing and impacting your mind, which can drive you to reactions and actions and behaviours that do not serve you for your highest good.

It is your mind that helps you make choices and decisions in life. It is your mind that moves between emotional states like fear and love, that creates peace and war. It is your mind that chooses which paths you take in life – a path of empowerment or a path of destruction, inside of you and out. And that is why your mind is sacred, and why it is important you ensure it is clean and pure.

Your mind is your holy space and connects you to life.

Your mind has the power to connect, create, influence and empower you. It also has the power to destroy and disempower you. You decide: which one are you?

Your entire life experience starts in the mind and then channels its way into your body, and then it manifests in the real world through reactions, actions and behaviours. This is not only for you, it is true for others in life too. Your mind, and the way you work with your experience and the way you set your mindset, is a choice. You decide.

The tools for working with your mental self

ACKNOWLEDGE

To acknowledge means to accept or admit the existence or truth of what is happening inside of your mind.

Always start with the truth. What is happening to you in your mind?

Acknowledge the truth

What am I seeing?

What am I hearing?

What am I feeling?

What am I perceiving?

What am I experiencing?

Acknowledge the mental state you are in.

Mental state

What mental state am I in?

Positive

Neutral

Negative

A positive mental state means it feels good in the mind.

A neutral mental state means it feels natural in the mind.

A negative mental state means it feels bad in the mind.

Once you have acknowledged your true mental state, you can start to work with your mind.

CLEAR YOUR MIND

A clear mind – free of clutter, chaos, noise, obstructions and intrusions – will allow you to step into alignment with your whole self.

When you are in alignment with your whole self (in harmony, in flow, in agreement with yourself and life), you will be able to connect to your whole self including your spirit.

A clear mind helps you to create space inside of yourself, which enables you to connect to your inner voice.

A clear mind helps you to maintain mental stillness and not get caught up in chaos and noise that unfolds with everyday life.

A clear mind helps you to connect with all parts of yourself and helps you to access your inner energy and strength.

Practice: Take time to create space.

Create space in your mind

To help you create space in your mind, limit:
- media and technology
- noise, chaos, conflict
- stirring beliefs, judgements, opinions or conclusions
- getting caught up in others' beliefs, judgements, opinions or conclusions

Practice: Ten minutes of silence

- Spend at least 10 minutes a day sitting in silence.
- Silence means no sound, no reaction, no action (inside and out).
- Allow yourself to simply be still in mind, body and spirit.
- Move your mind to a sacred space or a silent place.
- Set an alarm to signify the end of your practice, so you can fully let go and surrender for the duration.

This helps you to:
- clear an overactive mind and still a reactive body
- move stuck, repeated or reactive emotions and thoughts
- align with your whole self, and align with the spirit of life
- to your core.

EXERCISE: CREATE A SACRED SPACE

Close your eyes
Meet your mind
Meet your body
Breathe in and out
When you are ready, imagine a line appearing in your mind
This line is your sacred power
Slowly draw this line into a square
As you draw this line, know that
This line is creating a sacred space for you
Inside of this sacred space, nothing can touch you

Inside of this sacred space, you can be your whole self
Inside of this sacred space, you get to meet all of you
Inside of this sacred space, you surrender and let go
Inside of this sacred space, you are loved
<u>YOU ARE SAFE.</u>

This sacred space is always there, inside you, inside your mind, ready for you to enter.

CLEAN THE MIND

Each moment of your life is a chance for you to start fresh and lead from a pure place.

A clean mind – one not influenced, contaminated or poisoned from the past (or even yesterday), or influenced by what others say, or in a place where it is confused by senses – is a chance for you to make a choice and not allow the lingering emotions, thoughts or feelings of yesterday to influence your mind, or keep stirring in your mind, or impact you negatively.

Each moment of your life is a chance for you to start again in your mind in a new way, and from a clean and pure space.

Why clean the mind?

Imagine an overloaded, cluttered room that has been used for a lifetime of hoarding. What happens when you walk into a room like that and want to add more to it, but do not want to let go of what is already there? Is there space? Is there room to change or move? No – you have limited room to move or grow, and if you keep adding more, you will get stuck and blocked.

Practice: Clean the conscious mind

> Be present

Clean means your mind is pure and in the present.

> Am I in the present?
>
> Am I responding to the present only?

To help your conscious mind to stay clean and in the present moment, ask yourself:

Is my mind in the present or the past?

Am I responding in the present only?

Are my emotions and feelings mixed?

Practice: Clean the subconscious mind

To keep your mind pure and clean, use:

observation – a passive act to see what is happening to you in your mind

introspection – analysing and examining in detail, and explaining and interpreting

Also clear the following:

Old emotions and feelings connected to a past experience or memory can resurface and rise in you as you experience the present. This can impact your present state of mind, and you may react in the same way that you did in the past or may start to feel mentally and emotionally stuck in the same place.

To help you clear your subconscious mind, each moment an emotion arises, especially negative emotions, ask yourself:

> Is this emotion "old" or "new"?

Allow yourself to work with the emotion – see it, know it, understand it. (Use the Dictionary of Feelings to help you move these emotions from the dark inside of you out into the light so you can release them.)

Whether an emotion is being replayed by the past or present, a question to always ask yourself after you acknowledge the emotion is:

How do I react to this emotion?

Old thoughts will keep stirring or rising in your mind. As each thought arises, use observation and introspection. Then ask yourself:

Does this thought serve me?

Is this thought keeping me stuck in a mental cycle or circle?

Thoughts
"Do I need this thought?"

Old opinions based on your past events, positions, experiences and views will keep stirring inside of you, and you will keep reacting and acting from the same space, and this will influence and impact your mind.

Opinions
"Can I let go of this opinion?"

Old Conclusions – the mind has reached many **conclusions** to try and make sense of the world it is living in and experiencing.

Conclusions lead to **judgements**, and judgements can keep your mind blocked and stuck, as you have told your mind not to look beyond the conclusion. So before you reach a conclusion, ask yourself:

> Why am I making this conclusion?

Then ask yourself:

> Conclusions
>
> "Is this conclusion right?"

These two questions allow you to open up your mind beyond the conclusion.

Old judgements have been reached inside of you based on past experience. Time passes by, things change, but the judgement still resides in you, and your mind will use this to get in the way of your mental view. Before you judge, ask yourself:

> Why am I judging?

and ask:

Is this an old judgement made at a different time in my life?
Is it still true?
Do I have a new life view?
Pause before you judge, and ask yourself:

> Judgments
>
> Is this judgment justified?

Old beliefs – an acceptance of how something is – have been created inside of you based on a past experience.

Each time you react, act or behave according to a belief, ask:
Is this true?

Can I make room for new beliefs?

> Beliefs
>
> Is this belief still true?

Practice: How did I create this?

Revisiting chapters 1 and 2 will help you to go back to basics and understand how emotions, thoughts, feelings, beliefs, judgements, opinions and conclusions are created. When you lose your way, take your mind back to the basics of who you are and ask yourself:

How did I create this part of me?

Practice: Release what no longer serves you

It is time to **release** what no longer serves you in life – you need to clear what is inside of you so you can make room for something new, and open your mind to a new view.

Affirm: _I am ready to release_.

> I am ready to release what no longer serves me.

When you are ready:

Close your eyes

Breathe in

Breathe out

Feel life in your breath, and start to move your mind slowly into your whole being

Relax

When you feel aligned with your whole self, say in clear words:

I am ready to release what no longer serves me.

As you say this, a shift will happen inside of you. And next time something unhelpful arises in you, you will know what to do to release what no longer serves you.

You are now conscious and aware that this is not who you are anymore in the present moment in time – and you will mentally become aware that what is inside of you or rising inside of you no longer serves you and is holding you back. There will be no need to do anything, the shift will happen naturally with your spirit; it may start with a small internal movement or struggle, but you will start to notice a change. You may stop reacting in the same way, or the change can happen outside of you and you may stop acting a certain way – this creates space.

NB: There are many teachers worldwide specialized in helping clear the subconscious mind, so if you find you cannot do this alone, try to find a professional who can help you.

BREATHING – THE POWER OF BREATH

Your breath is your life-force energy; it has power and connects you to life. If your mind is always moving, overactive and constantly stirring emotions based on what it is experiencing through your physical senses, this means your mind is overworking and needs to rest. One way to help yourself mentally in the present moment is to take a moment for yourself, close your eyes and gently move your mental attention to your breath. As you do this, you allow your mind to rest and let the power that is your life breath take over. Your breath will help you move through stuck energy and emotions and thoughts that are stirring inside of you, and your breath will help you reconnect with your whole self and help you rebalance and be in alignment and harmony with yourself again.

> Breath is life.
>
> Inhale
> Exhale

Practice: Natural breathing

Gently and slowly inhale and exhale your breathing in a natural way.

Close your eyes
Breathe
Life
Inhale
Exhale
Naturally
Slowly

Allow your mind to follow your natural breath patterns that are connected to life. Your breath will have a rhythm and the rhythm will guide you.

Do not force, resist, struggle with or manipulate your breathing – allow it to be natural.

Practice: Deep breathing

Deeply inhale to your navel, hold in, then deeply exhale.

Close eyes
Breathe

Inhale through your nose

Deep

To

Navel

Hold as long as you can

Exhale through your mouth

Repeat five times

If you are feeling any stress, struggle, resistance, hurt or pain, breathe deeply into the negative space so you can relieve any pain, pressure, stress, hurt or resistance.

Allow yourself to be guided to a breathwork specialist, especially if you need help in releasing old emotions and feelings that are continuously stirring inside of you and take room, or if you need help healing old wounds that keep rising. Breathwork can help you release what is inside of you.

Breath
Use your breath to fully align.

Finally, use your breath to bring yourself back to you.

Other ways to help the mind

MEDITATION

Meditation can bring awareness, allowing you to mentally see, know and understand what is happening to you, inside of you and outside of you – to see deeply, beyond the layers.

The meditation style that aligns with this guide works with your mental and emotional states. This meditation style allows you to work with the emotions and feelings that naturally arise in you and reveal themselves to you instead of controlling, fighting with or managing your feelings, or instead of mentally controlling what you think you should feel, or instead of constantly searching for a sense of peace, joy or happiness.

Allow yourself to surrender to your truth and see where you are in your life right now. Allow your mind to guide you to the reality of your experience. Let your mental and emotional thoughts, feelings and sensations that have been stirring inside of you naturally rise to the surface so you can meet what is inside of you.

This natural meditation and awareness will help you to meet your mental and emotional states, and will help you understand what you are experiencing in life from your perspective, position and view.

Meet Your Emotions:

Fear

Anger

Anxiety

Depression

Grief

Hurt

Hate

Love

Joy

I am ready to meet you.

Warning: If you have experienced trauma or a really painful experience, you will need professional help and guidance to help you meet and move through painful mental and emotional states.

Practice: Meditation 1 – Meet your emotions

Meet your emotions as they come into creation and start to stir or enter your mind in the present moment.

To meditate in the present moment means to simply move your mind into a new space of awareness where you can observe and introspect, instead of being caught up in or reacting to what is happening to you. By gently moving your mind into a new area or space, you can see your whole self, inside and out.

In real time:

As an emotion arises in you

Instead of reacting to it

Step back from yourself

Move your mind into

Awareness mode

Observation mode

Introspection mode

Mentally see yourself (inside)

What is stirring?

Can you feel it?

Can you understand it?

It is forming into an emotion

What is this emotion?

Do you see it?

Do you know it?

Do you understand it?

Can you name it?

If not, focus on how you feel

How does your mind feel?

Good or bad?

How does your body feel?

Good or bad?

What are the symptoms of your experience?

Do you feel pleasant, comfortable?

Do you feel restless, discomfort?

If you feel discomfort

Breathe through where it feels uncomfortable

However, observe

How does your breath feel?

How does your heart feel?

How do your muscles feel?

How does your skin feel?

Bad, restless, uncomfortable?

Breathe life into those areas

Breathe through discomfort

Breathe through physical symptoms

Breathe through emotional experiences

Now, slowly move your mind outside

Observe your environment

Look around you

Where are you?

Who are you with?

What is happening?

Know you are safe.

As the emotions move through you, it is safe for you to move your mind back to a place where you can be fully present and interact again. You will know when the emotion has moved through you as your mind and body will move back into a homeostasis state – a state of balance. There will be no stirring or movement, it will be a natural, neutral state; your heartbeat and breathing is regulated and your muscles feel at ease and relax; your mind feels clear and your body is calm.

Meet your emotions meditation helps you to be aware of:

What the emotion is
The symptoms
Where you are
Who you are with
How you react
How you behave
How you feel

Practice: Meditation 2 - Reflect on your emotions

Look back at the emotions that passed through your mind and body over the course of the day.

At the end of your day
Before you sleep at night
Find a comfortable, safe space
Lie down
When you are ready
Close your eyes
Start to
Breathe in
Breathe out
Slowly
Relaxing
Surrendering
Mind
Body
To
Breath

When you are ready
In your own time
Place one hand gently on your stomach
Place another hand gently on your heart
Keep breathing
Naturally
In
Out
Keep eyes closed
Keep breathing

When you are ready
Gently move your mind back
To the beginning of your day
Where were you as you woke?
Where did you move to next?
What did you do in the day?
Who did you speak to?
What did you physically do?
How did events unfold for you?
How was your day?
Who did you interact with?
What emotions did you feel?
Did you feel good?
Did you feel bad?
If bad, where was your mind?
In the present, past or future?
How did you feel today?
Did your body relax?
Did your body become tense?
Could you see the emotions?

Were you aware of them?
How did you react to them?
Did you work with them?
Did you align with your truth?
Did your words match your truth?
Did your actions match your truth?
Are you revealing the whole truth?
Or are you working with half-truths?
Are you reacting to how it makes you feel inside?
Keep your eyes closed
Keep breathing
Keep your eyes closed
Keep reflecting

When you are ready
Slowly bring your mind back to the present moment
In mind
In body
Open your eyes
You are now back in the room, where you laid down

The **reflect on your emotions meditation** helps you to
be aware of:
What the emotion was
Where you were
Who you were with
How you reacted
How you behaved
How you felt

Practice: Meditation 3 – Who am I when I am with my emotions?

The goal of this meditation is to see your whole self clearly in the past and to see how you reacted when you met certain emotions and felt certain feelings – who did you become?

Find a comfortable, safe space
Allow yourself to lie down
When you are ready
Close your eyes
Breathe in,
Breathe out
Slowly
Relaxing
Surrendering
Mind
Body
To
Breath

When you are ready
In your own time
Remember a memory
A time when you felt strong emotions
Strong, uncomfortable emotions
Or strong, pleasant emotions
What was the event?
Who was there?
What was happening?
How did you feel?

How did you react?
How did you act?
Were you aligned?

Observe yourself
Ask:

Who am I?

Who am I when I meet Fear?
Who am I when I meet Anger?
Who am I when I meet Anxiety?
Who am I when I meet Hurt?
Who am I when I meet Hate?
Who am I when I meet Love?
Who am I when I meet Joy?

See who you are when you meet emotions. Start with negative emotions, and see how the discomfort, hurt or pain influences and impacts you, and so creates further and unnecessary conflict, hurt and pain. Then see who you are when you experience love, joy and happiness. Are you the same? Do you change when you feel hurt and pain?

NB: If you want to learn how to work with meditation, there are many teachers worldwide. Allow yourself to be guided to specialists who can teach you how to clear your mind and release emotions.

MINDFULNESS

To be mindful is to focus your awareness on the present moment rather than allowing your mind to move back and forth from the past into the present and the future.

Mindfulness helps you to surrender your entire being into the present moment of life. It allows you to be fully present in the moment. Wherever you are – at home or work, with loved ones or with others, attending to a task or relaxing – mindfulness allows you to step into your whole self, accept where you are and be there as a whole being. It allows you to see and experience the moment, instead of mentally wishing you were elsewhere, or resisting, pushing, forcing or detaching your mind, or only being half present. Mindfulness is a way of honouring your whole self, your whole life and your loved ones – knowing that, as life is unfolding in front of you, you are giving your entire being, including your mind, to the experience, and that you are doing your best to be where you are in your life. As life moves and changes and unfolds, you will know the truth is that you did your best.

Warning: Please note that being mindful does not apply to life-threatening or dangerous situations.

Mindful Acceptance
"I accept where I am."

MINDFUL ACCEPTANCE

Accepting where you are in the moment.

When you mentally accept where you are in the moment, you surrender your mind and body to the present moment without feeling the need to fight or struggle or push or resist.

Mindful acceptance frees up energy and space in your mind so you can stop fighting and struggling and get the help you need. It also frees up the space your mind uses when it feels it should be elsewhere and your body is restless and not fully present in the moment. You can use this free space to see where you are in your life, know the truth of how you feel, and find new ways, new choices and decisions that can help empower you.

NB: If you are experiencing dark thoughts or painful emotions, or if someone is treating you in an unacceptable way, accepting the moment and accepting what is happening will help you to get the help that you need; it will help you to find a way and heal. There is help for you if you need it.

Practice: Affirmation

Say to yourself:

> I am where I am.

It is easy for you to surrender and accept the moment in your mind if you can remember moments are not static – they move and change.

Practice: Mindful alarm

Mindful alarms help bring your mind back to the present moment if it has wandered into the past or future.

Set an alarm for every 30 or 60 minutes.

When the alarm rings, ask yourself:

> Where is my mind?

Practice: Mindful chores

Household chores can be the source of much mental conflict, and can impact your state of the mind if they are not done when or in the way your mind expects them to be done, either by yourself or another person. Chores can instantly place your mind into a negative state. Annoyance, irritation and frustration can build up and lead to anger and rage. The expectations of chores break the harmony in households. It is important you create a home where there is mental space for yourself and others to feel comfortable.

Mindful chores help you to create energy and space in your home and help you appreciate your life and home. They can help you to step outside of your mind and be present in your daily life, while at the same time help you to appreciate your home, that sacred space that your mind and body physically lives in.

Mindful Chores

"I choose to be out of my mind and into my life."

Spend 30 minutes a day mindfully:

- making the bed
- washing up
- doing laundry
- hoovering and dusting
- tidying up

Do the above without noise or interruptions, making sure your mind is fully present in the activities.

Allowing yourself and each person in your home to be mindful of chores and tasks helps yourself and others; it is a simple act of mental kindness as you choose to step into the physical world without and reconnect fully with life.

As you do your chores, notice where you are, what you have in life, and who you are with. Be present in your life in that moment.

As you take time to prepare food, allow space in your mind to appreciate the food you have. Allow yourself mental space to prepare food and eat the food you have made, and feel appreciation that you can do this.

Allow yourself to be present.

MINDFUL COMMUNICATION

Mindful communication allows you to align your words with your truth, to speak words that match the way you think and feel in your mind and body. This helps you to release the unseen parts of you that are stirring inside of you via language and communication.

Make sure you use words that explain **clearly** what you are experiencing.

Practice: Mindful communication – I am

As you communicate, start with _I am_, and then explain what your senses experience.

```
Mindful Communication

I am Seeing
I am Hearing
I am Feeling
I am Thinking
I am Perceiving
I am Experiencing
```

Practice: Mindful communication – inside out

This is a way for you to find the words that can help you explain the unseen, unrevealed and unspoken parts of you.

If you start to communicate from the inside outwards, this can help you release the truth of what is happening to you inside – your emotions, feelings, thoughts.

Explain what you are experiencing **inside**:

I am seeing... inside
I am hearing... inside
I am feeling... inside
I am thinking... inside
I am perceiving... inside
I am experiencing... inside

This can help you build a bridge over the gap formed by misunderstanding, miscommunication and lies, and can prevent you from blaming or shaming another person.

Practice: Mindful communication – speak your truth

The truth means how it is for you.

Ensure your words **align** with the truth of what you are experiencing – do not lie, hide, deny or dismiss the truth.

```
Mindful Communication
Do these words align with the truth?
```

Use words to fully explain what you are seeing, hearing, thinking, perceiving and experiencing:

I am seeing… Speak your truth.
I am hearing… Speak your truth.
I am feeling… Speak your truth.
I am thinking… Speak your truth.
I am perceiving… Speak your truth.
I am experiencing… Speak your truth.

Don't forget about what is happening in the space in between where the unexpressed, unspoken and unseen emotions, thoughts and feelings lie. Try and find a way to explain these.

I am seeing… in the space in between. *Speak your truth.*
I am experiencing… in the space in between. *Speak your truth.*
I am feeling… in the space in between. *Speak your truth.*
I am thinking… in the space in between. *Speak your truth.*
I am perceiving… in the space in between. *Speak your truth.*

Or, if this does not feel comfortable for you, simply start the truth with:

> I am sensing

Then reveal in words what you are **aware** of your mind and body experiencing.

> It is in my awareness

MINDFUL EATING

Being mindful about eating allows you to mentally focus on the food you prepare and eat in the present moment of life. It allows your senses to fully immerse in the experience and helps you to connect with and enjoy life.

> Mindful Eating
> "How does my food smell?"
> "How does my food taste?"

Think about whether you really:
   See your food
   Enjoy your food
   Appreciate your food.

MINDFUL HABITS

Habits are repeated actions that can be mental or physical.

As you move through life and fall into repeated actions and habits, or react and act automatically or unconsciously, every now and then pause and ask yourself:

Why am I doing this?

It is in this pause and in the asking of the question that you create the space in your mind to be able to make a new choice or decision; it is here that you create change.

Mindful Habits

"Why am I doing this?"

MINDFUL MOMENTS

Mindful moments allow your mind to be fully present so you can immerse yourself into the experience of your life; you can notice the little things you normally take for granted.

Practice: Mindful moments

Stop what you are doing and say:

I am in the present moment.

Mindful Moments

"I am in the present moment."

If your mind still wanders, use your five senses to experience the present moment fully. Say where you are and name five things around you:

I am...
I can see...
I can hear...
I can smell...
I can taste...
I can touch...

Five senses:

I see

I hear

I smell

I taste

I touch

MINDFUL LISTENING

When you listen mindfully, you give your entire mental attention to another person as they communicate with you. Mindful listening allows you to fully connect with another person without creating interruptions in your mind, which can block you from fully connecting. When you mindfully listen, you give your mind a rest, and as you rest your mind, you open yourself and your hearing and other senses to another human being, which allows you to fully connect with the other person and allow the other person to be fully seen and heard.

Mindful listening improves connection, communication, understanding and compassion.

Mindful Listening

- Listen without assumption.

- Listen without criticism.

- Listen without judgment.

- Listen without interruption.

Practice: Mindful listening

Listen without the need to immediately express a view.

Listen without blocking, assumption, criticism, judgement or interruption.

MINDFUL TASKS

Mindful tasks help you to step outside of your mind and be fully present in your daily tasks.

Mindful Tasks

"I give my full attention to this task."

If you have to leave a task half-finished – perhaps because you do not have time to finish the task or need to come back to it at a later point – when you move your attention away from the task, fully let go. Just come back to it when you are ready, and approach it mindfully again.

MINDFUL TRUTH

Take a moment to pause and ask yourself a question to connect to your truth.

In life you will lose your way many times over as you make your way through phases, stages, events and circumstances of life. There will be times on your life journey when your mental and emotional states will get in the way. There will be times when your mind and body will push you and test you and move you through painful and uncomfortable negative states that cause extreme discomfort; this can change you as you mentally try and find your way through, and you feel as if you are moving far away from yourself. It can be easy to lose yourself through layers of negative emotions. You may start to react and act and behave in ways that do not align with your truth. This is why it is essential to stay close to your truth so you can stay close to you. Each time you struggle or feel emotional pain, before you react and act and behave, ask yourself:

Mindful Truth
"Am I being true to myself or others?"

If the answer is <u>Yes</u>, then you are working with your truth; if it is <u>No</u>, then you are not being entirely true to yourself.

If the answer is <u>No</u>, what is happening to you to cause this? Are you blocking, hiding, denying, dismissing, resisting, pushing, ignoring or fighting with parts of yourself, inside or out?

Moving the mind: Do not Stay stuck

MIND SHIFT

A mind shift is a mental movement that allows you to get out of a mental rut. It helps you move your mind to a new space where you can change your mental experience, your focus, or your perception so you can experience something positive, neutral or new again.

If you are mentally struggling and in pain and have been in the same mental place for a long time, one of the ways to help you to ease your struggle and pain is for you to shift your mind into a new space or new direction that can help you to find new ways of being. Being in a new space mentally can help you to surrender, to let go of the pain, struggle and resistance, even for a moment. Mind shifts can help you to see life through a new lens, or feel an emotion that you have not felt in a long time.

MIND SHIFT – AFFIRMATION

An affirmation is a creation of strong, powerful words created to help empower your mind. An affirmation can create space for positive words in your mind. Affirmation, if practised healthily and successfully, can help calm and strengthen the mind. An affirmation can help shift your mind from a place of chaos, clutter, disturbance and struggle toward a position of strength and empowerment. The words created in an affirmation can help you to feel powerful; these words can support you, uphold you and empower you.

It is important that affirmations do not mask the truth of how you feel. First, acknowledge and work with the truth of how you feel, and then start to gather words to help you.

Practice: Make a powerful statement

Choose clean, clear, powerful words that match with the truth of how you want to feel. What are these powerful words you want to say and confirm to yourself?

If you feel comfortable, look at yourself in the mirror as you speak these words.

Alternatively, close your eyes, put your hand on your heart and say the words with pure intention.

Affirmation:

"I am a healthy mind."

"I am a healthy body."

"I am a healthy mind."

"I am a healthy body."

(repeat x 8 times)

MIND SHIFT – APPRECIATION

Move your mind to a place where you can see and feel and recognize the value in your life.

Appreciation is a deep healing method that can help you transform your inner mind. If you are struggling in life, appreciation can help shift your mind from that dark place where you cannot see or think clearly to a new place that has light. Appreciation can help you to gently release and let go of negative emotions that are stirring inside of you and which keep you in a dark place. A deep moment of appreciation will help you to unblock stuck or suppressed energy; it can help you to stop resisting or fighting or going deeper within yourself to a darker place. Appreciation can help you see new things that are otherwise missed if you are stuck in a dark place.

Appreciation
What do I truly appreciate?

EXERCISE: TO HELP YOU FIND APPRECIATION

Appreciation connects you to the roots of positive emotions: joy, unconditional love.

Appreciation

Close your eyes

Place your hand on your heart

Take five deep breaths

Inhale

Exhale

Move mind to breath

When ready

Ask Questions

What do I appreciate in life?

Allow the words to flow to you

Can you name three?

You are now in appreciation mode. This simple act moves your mind and body into a place and space of appreciation.

MIND SHIFT – GRATITUDE

Feeling grateful in life comes from deep within you – it is your truth of how you feel about life.

Gratitude

"What am I truly and deeply grateful for?"

Finding a way to feel grateful about something will help you mentally move away from uncertainty. To feel grateful from a true place, it is important you align your mind and body and spirit with your whole self and life.

You can feel grateful just for the experience of living and experiencing life – this opens up your mind to move and connect to life, and at the root of this is joy and unconditional love.

Practice: To help you find gratitude

Close your eyes
Place your hand on your heart
Ask:
What am I deeply grateful for?

If you are struggling to see, think or feel anything, keep a **gratitude journal** – a log book in which you keep a note of all the grateful times in life.

MIND SHIFT – INSPIRATION

Inspiration is the process of being mentally stimulated in a positive way and in a way that connects you to your whole self and creation and life.

Inspiration
What inspires me?

EXERCISE: TRY A NEW WAY OF BEING

One of the most healing ways for you to be mentally stimulated and inspired is for your mind to let go of thinking, fixing and feeling – just immerse yourself in living and being and enjoying life.

Have a go at a new activity and see where it leads you. This could be anything pure and simple that allows you to connect to your spirit, such as:

Art

Colours

Cooking

Dancing

Painting

Singing

Music

Nature

MIND SHIFT – JOY

Joy is the natural state you were in when you first came to life, when you were born. It is a state that connects you to life and that helps you to connect to your whole being. If you are experiencing negative emotions day after day and cannot find joy, remember it is always within you. Joy lies beneath all of your life experiences and emotions. When you are ready to reconnect with joy, it will reveal itself to you.

Practice: To help you find joy

Close your eyes

Open your mind and other senses

Place your hand on you heart
Ask yourself:
When was the last time I felt joy?

Joy
"When do I feel pure joy?"

If you cannot answer this, take your mind back in time. When you were a child and day-to-day life had not taken over, it was probably easier for you to find joy and wonder in the simpler things in life, so open your mind and ask yourself:

Joy
What five things gave me joy as a child?

Keep an open mind, and allow yourself to help you remember that joy again.

Or, think of a time when you gave joy to someone and saw their eyes and their smile – how did that make you feel?

When you connect to a joyful memory – especially a childhood one when it was easier to fall into alignment with life and your whole self – positive emotions will stir, and these positive memories can help move your mind and body back into a positive state.

MIND SHIFT – EQUANIMITY
Equanimity is a mental state that is undisturbed by emotion and experience. It is a state of mind that helps you to keep your mind and body balanced, especially during hard, dark, difficult, turbulent and painful times. It is easier for you to see and think

clearly in a state of equanimity. To help your mind to move into this neutral state, you first need to understand equanimity.

Equanimity

Life's nature is impermanence

It is the essence of life that things shift, change and grow – nothing in life stays as it is. Understanding human nature and life and learning to let go of your mental experiences will bring you equanimity, allowing your mind to move with life. Life's nature is impermanence – nothing is entirely still or stuck – there is always some movement or development. As such, it is not natural in life to hold on to things, as life moves and flows. Being in a state of equanimity means you allow your mind, body and spirit to flow and change with these life changes.

Equanimity

Let go of resistance and clinging

Practice: Observe and let go

Equanimity is a mental act and a personal choice. It is an act of letting go and surrendering – not holding on to what you are experiencing in your mind. This means you do not repeat what you need to let go, and you do not resist the process of letting go.

Allow your energy, emotions, thoughts and narrative to appear

Observe your energy, emotions, thoughts and narrative

Let go of your energy, emotions, thoughts and narrative

Practice: Affirmation – This time will soon pass

If you are struggling or working against yourself and life, or you feel mentally stuck or blocked, remember it does not have to stay this way – you can move through what you are experiencing. Open your mind to move to a state of equanimity and return to nature's ways.

Affirmation: *This time will pass. This is not permanent.*

These words will allow you to let go, allow room for gentle mental movement and change, and help you let go of the ways that you hold on to experiences in your mind.

MIND SHIFT – NARRATIVE

Be aware of the negative words or negative story that you form in your mind, and take steps to change or erase the narrative.

Move away from the story stuck in your mind to help you create space for yourself and to allow room for a new view, a new perspective or a new way of feeling.

Narrative

"What is the story in my mind?"

"How long has this story been in my mind?"

"Is the story the entire truth, or my truth?"

"How can I change this story?"

Practice: Erasing a stuck narrative from your mind

How many times have your emotions, feelings and thoughts led to a negative story that takes up a lot of your mind space? How many times has your mind filled up with:

Assumptions

Expectations

What if… ?

Watch Out!

Worst-case scenario

A victim story

A negative story

A blame story?

Where has this mental activity led you? How many times has it led you into a negative state, stirring up old emotions and wounds from the past? The best way to mentally shift from a negative space is to change the narrative in your mind.

To do this, when you start to be aware of a story, take a mental action:

Say, **"Stop."**

Imagine yourself erasing your negative mental narrative, like a rubber removes pencil.

Practice: Naked narrative

Expose your mental narrative – take it out from the dark and into the light, exposing it for you to clearly see. Make your narrative naked.

Naked narrative: What was happening in my mind?

MIND SHIFT – PERCEPTION

Change your perception, and see in a new way.

> Find your power through perception

Revisit chapter 2 for more details on perception, but here is a quick reminder.

In life your mind and body will be placed in a
Position (the place where you are and where you stand)
From your position, your mind and body will have a
Viewpoint
From this viewpoint, your mind and body will have a
View
From this view, your mind will create a
Perception (using your senses to understand and interpret what you experience)
From your perception you will gain a
Perspective (a particular way of viewing something, a point of view)
And it is from your perspective that you will start to experience
Emotions (an experience in your mind that moves it into a state: good, neutral or bad)
Those emotions will transfer to your physical body and be felt as
Feelings (an experience in your mind that moves into a state: good, neutral or bad)

Over time, all that you experience in life will be filtered through your:

Life lens (a lens you view life through)

World view (your perception of your world – inside and out)

Once you understand perception, ask yourself:

> Through which lens am I experiencing life?

Are you experiencing life through the lens of love?
Are you experiencing life through the lens of fear?

If you are experiencing repeated negative emotions inside of you, somehow, somewhere, you are stuck in fear or sadness. Underneath all emotional pain and suffering are the negative emotion roots of fear and sadness. This root emotion will cloud your life lens and means you will be seeing and experiencing life through the lens of fear or sadness.

A CLOUDED LIFE LENS

A **clouded life lens** means your view on life is no longer clear and pure and purely in the present moment; rather, it is clouded by how you are feeling on the inside. Repeated negative emotions trapped inside of you from your past experiences will cloud your life lens and when life takes a bad turn you will start to struggle and have a pessimistic view.

If fear influences and clouds your life lens, you will not feel safe. You will not trust what is happening to you, which will stir other negative emotions that impact on your body. If this is how it feels in your mind right now, it is time to clean your life lens, so you can start to relook at and experience life differently.

Practice: Clean your life lens

A clean and clear life lens helps you to experience life purely in the present moment and helps your mind and body to connect to life in the present moment. It gives you new insights on life, a new way of understanding life, and helps you to move through life in the present moment alone, day by day. When your lens is clean and clear, it is not influenced or distorted or clouded by yesterday, and this can help you to feel free in mind and body.

To help you clean your life lens, start with the following practices:

Clear your mind – Be still

Clear your mind – Sit for ten minutes in silence

Clear your mind – Create a sacred space in your mind

Clean your conscious mind – Experience your life in the present moment only

Clean your sub-conscious mind – Release what no longer serves you will on the inside of you

Work "with" your negative emotions – Acknowledge them, use the Dictionary of Feelings

Meditate – Meet your emotions – See what happens when you meet emotions.

Meditate – Who am I? – Reflect on how negative emotions change your life and lens.

Mindshift – Joy – Move your mind to a place and time of joy. What gave you joy as a child?

Mind Shift – Equanimity – Move your mind to a state of equanimity; a neutral place where you can see clearly.

As you start the process of being aware of what is happening inside you and realize that your past is influencing your present, take steps to start to work with your emotions and feelings, instead of ignoring them or burying them and reacting from them.

Work with them and release them inside of you, or move them from a dark place into the light. Doing this will help to clear your life lens, and you will start to experience:

A new life lens.

Warning: Do not do this without professional help or professional guidance, it is important you get help.

EXERCISE: REVISIT AND RELOOK

Another way to help you change your perception is to take a mental and/or physical journey and revisit or relook at a time or place in your life that impacted your state of mind. With the help of a professional, find a way to revisit the situation, circumstances and events. The goal of reviewing event(s) is to face and accept and acknowledge what has happened to you, but from a perspective that you are now where you are – you got through it, you survived, you had the power to survive. In time, you will be able to see this and feel it, so work through the negative emotions that are now inside of you and keeping you stuck. As they rise inside of you so they can be seen, you will have the strength to do the work inside of you; and when you do, you will find the power to take off the old lens, as you will know you no longer need to experience life through this lens which is holding you back.

Remember, always take a moment to ask:
Which lens am I experiencing my life through – love or fear?

MIND SHIFT – PERSPECTIVE

You may need to change your perspective, i.e., your position and view, if you feel mentally stuck and as though your life is moving around in circles, repeating the same internal pain again and again; if it feels, no matter how hard you try, that your mind constantly repeats the same negative emotions and feelings; or if you are constantly and consistently experiencing:

Mental disruption,

Mental resistance,

Mental discomfort,

Mental confusion and

Mental conflicts.

This negative cycle is a clear sign that something needs to change inside of you. You need to relook at your life or the situation you are in from a whole new perspective.

```
Perspective:
Change your position
Change your view
```

Practice: Mentally change your position and view

What is happening to you in your life? What is causing you to feel this mental, emotional pain? Choose an event or situation you are struggling with.

Where are you?

Who is involved?

Now mentally change your view.

Imagine you are no longer in your mind and body; instead you have stepped outside your mind and body and moved to a higher place to look down at the situation – a helicopter view.

You can now see all views, from all positions, and see everything that is happening from all points of view.

Do you see something new?

If this is hard for you to do, especially if there are events or other people involved and you cannot manage to see the situation from another person's point of view, try another way:

Put yourself in their life shoes.

Place yourself in a grounded position and place yourself in their shoes, in their mind and body – even if you detest them, you are now them, and they are you. What do you see? What do you feel? Is there something you didn't know or feel or understand when you were not in their shoes?

Or, if you still see nothing new or feel nothing new, try a new way – **understanding**. Understanding is the highest of views.

Find a new way to understand.

Move your mind higher and higher and higher, until you are in the most elevated position of all – as if you are the creator of all life. You can now see all of life and all life views. From here you will see something you could not see or understand or feel before – you can see how you react, act and function from a place only you know about, and therefore you can see that everyone else also reacts, acts and functions from a place only they know about. We all operate from a place based on our individual life journeys, from past experiences and emotions, from a place of passed-down teachings. We all operate from the only place we know.

Now that you see this, and now that you have gained this new understanding, which is the deepest understanding of all, do you have a new perspective?

Practice: Evolved perspective

An evolved perspective is one that has developed over time.

Sometimes there are no answers for why life happens, but if you live through mental and emotional pain, you can learn and evolve from these emotions and feelings, and you can release yourself from them so you can grow through life and see life from an evolved perspective.

The experience, emotions and feelings of past events are stuck inside you and keep rising to cause you double pain in real-time. Do not react to these rising emotions; instead, pause, create space, and stop seeking answers on the outside. It is time to look at yourself on the inside – ask yourself what is repeating inside of you, again and again,

What am I experiencing?
What am I thinking?
What am I feeling?
What words am I creating?

See if you can find a shared link – the same emotion or feeling that keeps repeating, the exact trigger that keeps repeating. Ask yourself:

What can I do to evolve here?
What am I not seeing?

Is there a way you can change your view:

mentally – change the way your mind sees the experience

emotionally – release the negative emotions inside of you

physically – place yourself in another person's shoes

spiritually – apply unconditional love to the experience

MIND SHIFT – VISUALIZATION

Visualization means to create a mental image.

If you are struggling, and your mind is resisting, fighting, or not in alignment or harmony, a simple practice to help you ease your mind is to visualize what you want and need in life, even if it seems far away and out of reach. Visualization will help you step into alignment with your entire being and, for a moment, allow you to stop struggling or being in disharmony. To help you with creating this vision, instead of forcing yourself to visualize it, the first question you need to ask your mind is:

What do I want?

Only after you are completely clear about what you want can you open your mind to find out if you can see it and believe it. As long as what you want is pure and from the heart, you can open your mind to visualize anything. Do not push your mind – allow what you want to be naturally seen. It may be helpful if you close your eyes, affirm what you want, and ask your mind:

Can I visualize this?

Visualization works much more powerfully when you are clear about what you want.

Practice: Visualize your future self

One way to help you mentally move into a new space and place is to use the power of visualization. Start to visualize your future self – how you want to be, how you want to look and feel.
　Start engaging in a daily visualization routine:

Morning: 15 minutes
Evening: 15 minutes

What do I want?
Close your eyes
Breathe
Inhale
Exhale
Align with
Your mind
Your body
Your spirit
Start to feel the power of your mind
Allow the power of your mind to create a vision

Use your imagination
Who do you want to be?
How do you want to feel?
What do you want to experience?
How do you want to be living your life?
Where do you want to be?

Feel all the emotions that come with your vision:
Happiness

Hope

Joy

Unconditional love

As you practise visualizing your future self, your mind should become unstuck and move slowly through the dark clouds, and through the repeated negative thoughts or emotions that have been keeping you stuck in fear and sadness and getting in the way of hope, joy and love.

MIND SHIFT – SURRENDER

Stop resisting, and surrender.

Practice: Let it go

Whatever you are experiencing in your mind, allow it to be and then gracefully let it go.

Do not force yourself to control or push your emotions.

Do not react to what is happening to you.

Give your mind a chance to rest.

Allow your mind to align with your body and spirit to find space for new ways.

Close your eyes, and say:

I let go.

Or simply say:

I surrender.

If you feel an internal struggle or resistance, or start to feel unsafe, reassure yourself that this surrender is just for a moment, just for a day, and allow yourself to surrender.

How does it feel?

MENTAL BLOCKS

Mental blocks stop you from tapping into or reaching your full attention.

Mental Block

"Why can I NOT do this?"

Mental Block

"What is holding me back?"

Practice: Ask questions

Why can I NOT do this?
What is holding me back?
Why is my mind blocked?

Ask your inner self for a reveal.
Close your eyes. Ask:
Reveal to me what is mentally holding me back

Open your mind and body to receive an answer.
Trust in that it will be revealed to you naturally when the time is right.

An answer should reveal itself to you in the coming days. When it does, it will feel like an epiphany – a moment of realization, a sense of knowingness, a moment of truth.

If you do not want to wait for a reveal, ask more questions to search inside yourself:

What is blocking me?
Is it an emotion? (Fear)
Is it a thought?
Is it a feeling?
Is it a belief?
Is it a judgement?
Is it a mindset?
Is it self-doubt?
Is it an excuse (locked in fear)?

MIND STILLNESS

Mind stillness is when you do not make any mental moves, reactions, or create any further motion in your mind.

> I will create no further motion

Practice: Mental stillness – sound meditation

Mental stillness can be achieved by using sound or vibration to clear your mind and bring your mind back into alignment with your whole self, or to place yourself into a deep meditative state.

Types of sound or vibration:
Tongue drum

Crystal bowls
Falling water
Raindrops
Ocean waves
Forest noises
Music (no vocals)

Sound therapy and sound meditation are healing for the mind and can help you move through blockages. They can move your mind out of a negative state and into a neutral or positive state. Any form of music that allows your mind to rest is healing.

The struggling mind – how to successfully work "with" mental pain

MENTAL ADDICTION
Addiction is when you cannot stop or do not want to stop. It is a repeated action that makes you feel you need something. The action is mental, emotional and physical, and can block you spiritually. A discovery process will help you see and understand the moment that led you to this place.

Addiction

Am I following a family pattern?
Is this who I am?
Who can I be without this?

Through this discovery process you can create a space for yourself and create a chance to make a choice and a change. You learn who you are, you discover the truth of who you are, deep down in your core. And you gain the power to let go of anything that is not serving you.

EXERCISE: WHAT IS A 12-STEP PROGRAMME?

A 12-step programme helps you to:

Forgive yourself and let go

Surrender to a higher power

Align with your whole self

Learn to live a new life without abusing and hurting yourself

Take the time to find out what a 12-step programme is, and how moving forward in 12 steps can help you to empower yourself as you move away from abuse, want, need or hurt.

MENTAL PRESSURE

Pressure is a state of mind and being that makes you feel as if someone or something is pushing you mentally, emotionally or physically with a sense of urgency or a high demand.

In life there is so much pressure.

Mental pressure
Body pressure
Education pressure
Career pressure
Family pressure

Life pressure
Peer pressure
Societal pressure
Self-pressure
World pressure

If you are experiencing pressure based on what the world wants you to be:

> Reset your mind

And, allow yourself to:

> Connect to your spirit

This should help you fully align to your life and whole self.

Note: See Chapter 12, *"How to work successfully with your spiritual self"*, for more guidance on how to relieve pressure.

MENTAL STRESS

Stress is a state of mind and being where you are experiencing a mental, emotional and/or physical strain and tension.

If you are feeling mental pressure, allow yourself to:

> Step into alignment with your whole self

Surrender, so you can step into alignment with your whole self and life.

Alternatively, there are holistic healing methods that can help you during stressful periods.

- Acupuncture
- Holistic massage
- Energy work

Holistic practitioners help relieve the stress inside your mind and body.

Take a look at "Stress" in the Dictionary of Feelings. Long-term stress can harm mind and body, and if you internalize the stress, it can impact your internal systems and lower your immune system.

MENTAL TRAUMA

Trauma is a deeply distressing or disturbing experience.

After a traumatic experience, it can be hard for you to trust life again or for your mind and body to feel safe again. If you do not feel safe, your mind will be in a constant state of fear, and your brain will be on high alert, scanning for a potential threat or danger; there may be unprocessed emotions and feelings that you are not ready to face or deal with. However, if you do not help yourself and work with the emotions and feelings that are stirring inside of you or if your trauma is not processed healthily, it can trap itself in your mind and body. As time moves on, your energy, emotions, thoughts and sensation memories attached to the trauma can start revealing themselves to you in a way that can haunt you or distort your world view. If you want to start to work with your trauma, there are three steps to take.

1. Acknowledge

The only way to heal from trauma is for you to acknowledge the truth of your experience.

What happened to you?

Is it still impacting you?

Is the trauma still inside your mind and body? Does it influence you and impact you every day?

Are you aware of it and how it affects you?

When you are ready to, affirm this truth:

I acknowledge the truth of my experience. It is still with me.

2. Accept

Once you have acknowledged your trauma, you need to accept that this has happened to you.

When you are ready to, affirm this truth:

I accept this happened to me.

3. Heal

Consider where in your mind and body this trauma impacts you. Ask yourself:

Am I ready to heal?

Only when you acknowledge the truth of your experience and can see that the trauma you have experienced is still in you and hurting you, causing you pain and holding you back in life, and only when you can accept the truth that this has happened to you can you open your mind to be ready to heal.

When you are ready to, look yourself in the eye, and affirm this truth:

I am ready to heal.

When you are ready to heal, I would advise you to turn to a professional who specializes in trauma and will be able to guide you through the emotions, thoughts and feelings attached to your trauma.

The Dictionary of Feelings will help you understand the emotions and feelings connected to the memory and the triggers. Look up "Trauma" to help you understand what is happening to you inside of you.

Sound meditation will also help you to release painful emotions inside of you; singing bowls and tongue drums create great sounds for helping you to step inside of your whole self and find power.

MENTAL OPPRESSION

Mental oppression is the experience of painful emotions you cannot express. It comes from the pressure and stress of your position in life and the way others see you and treat you because of this. If you are born into a home or into a society that you treats you or sees you as "less than", allow your mind to see all that you are, and more.

Hold your head high.
Be proud of who you are.
Know who you are in this life.

Do not allow the outside world to get you down. If you wake up every day feeling the world has a view on you and sees you in a certain way, and that you feel restricted, trapped and unable to change what is happening as it is too big for you, you can change yourself. You do not need to change yourself at your core, rather you can change the way you view your experience. Find the power from within to change this view, and step into your whole self and step into alignment with life. Inside you, there is the courage, joy and confidence you were born with; you are what you are, and be proud of it.

Practising affirmations can help you to move your state in to power, but only once you have acknowledged and accepted the truth of your experience. (Revisit Mind shift – Perception and Mind shift – Perspective.)

When you are ready, affirm:
I am who I am.
I am proud of who I am.

MENTAL PAIN

Mental pain is an uncomfortable, hurtful, unpleasant or painful sensation caused by experiences, emotions, thoughts, feelings, events, situations and circumstances in life. It is part of the human experience and affects everyone. As human beings, we all experience pain and hurt and suffer in some way or form.

Practice: How can I heal mental pain?

Close your eyes.
Speak to your inner self. (This connects you to your intuition and whole self.)
Ask:
How can I heal this pain?
Who can I turn to?

Is there someone you trust and admire – a loved one, a friend, a family member, a mentor? Speaking your truth to a friend is a great way for you to relieve the burden and pressure of life. Allow yourself to be helped, particularly when you need it most, just as you would do for others. This is life, and you are in it together with others, so use each other to heal your pain.

MENTAL CHECK-IN

Now that you are an adult, you get to make your own choices and decisions in life. You get to decide who you want to be and how you want to be. One of the best ways to ensure you are okay is for you to act like your very own parent and check in on yourself.

You have mentally experienced and been through lot in life, so check in on yourself as you need to be seen, heard and loved.

EXERCISE: CHECK IN ON YOURSELF

Close your eyes

See your inner child

See your inner teenager

See your struggling adult self

Ask yourself:

- Am I safe?
- What do I need?
- How can I help myself?

Finally, you have the power inside of you to say:

I got you.

The mind–body connection

The mind–body connection links one to another. Your mind impacts your body, your body feels the weight of your mind. It is important to understand the mind–body connection as it is very strong. Clearing and cleaning your mind is essential for a healthy body.

10

HOW TO SUCCESSFULLY WORK WITH YOUR EMOTIONAL SELF

Step 4: Learn how to work "with" and not "against" your emotions.

Emotional self

Your emotions and feelings are extremely influential in how you experience your life in your mind and body. Your emotions and feelings condition your mind and body and move your mind and body in and out of conditions and states. Your emotions and feelings have a huge impact on how you view life, interact with life and connect with life. Your emotions and feelings are intertwined and interconnected and connected to your mind, to your body, to your spirit, to your senses, and drive your reactions and actions and behaviours. Your emotions and feelings all start with energy.

Energy is the electrical impulses and magnetic waves that vibrate through your brain and body, as well as through the earth, the trees, the rivers, the universe. Energy connects you to life, and aligns you to the flow and the movement of life.

Emotions occur when your mind becomes aware of moving energy. The energy will start to stir in your mind and channel its way to your body. This moving energy is known as an emotion. This energy in motion will channel toward your body to drive you to react and act. It becomes a feeling.

Feelings are physical sensations, vibrations or triggers in the body. Feelings will rise in your whole body or in different parts of your body and will place your mind and body into an emotional state.

Emotional states are the condition your mind and body are in; they can be fleeting or more long-lasting. They can be positive, neutral or negative (see the Dictionary of Feelings).

The purpose of emotions and feelings

To connect you with others.
To protect and keep you safe from harm and danger.
To drive you toward making choices and decisions.

The way you feel in your mind and body will drive you in a certain direction. Your emotions and feelings will influence in which direction you take your life.

A simple universal law in life is this:
If something makes you feel **positive**, you are more likely to be drawn towards it – to want to experience it, be open to connecting with it, and trust in and feel safe. The root emotions are joy and unconditional love.

If something makes you feel **negative**, you are more likely to be drawn away from it – to not want to experience it, withdraw from it, mistrust it and feel unsafe. The root emotions are fear and sadness.

What influences your emotions/feelings?

Your emotions/feelings are influenced and impacted by your:

Mind: The way you acknowledge your emotions and feelings.

Body: The way you process your emotions and experience.

Experiences: Events, circumstances, situations, outcomes (past or present).

Perception: The way you understand through your senses (past or present).

Perspective: The way you view from your position (past or present).

Senses: The way you see, hear, smell, touch, taste (past or present).

Thoughts: A formation of words in your mind (past or present).

And further by your:

Beliefs: An acceptance of how something is, its truth (from past and present).

Conclusions: Decisions reached (from past and present).

Opinions: A personal view formed into the mind (from past and present).

Judgements: To come to a final conclusion on how something is (from past and present).

Narrative: A mental story that is created in your mind (from past and present).

Teachings: Ideas, knowledge, facts, taught by others (from past and present).

Handling your emotions/feeling

The **natural way** of dealing with your emotions is to **let go** of them, so they **flow** through your mind and body, and **release** outside of yourself so you are **free** of them.

The **unnatural way** of dealing with your emotions is to **hold on** to them, so they **block** your mind and body, and become **stuck** inside you.

The emotional struggle

Many people struggle with their emotions, and you too may struggle to:

Understand the emotions in your mind and the feelings in your body

Identify the emotions in your mind and the feelings in your body

Name the emotions your mind and the feelings in your body

Feel what you are feeling, or accept and acknowledge those feelings

Find the right **words** to match your emotions and feelings

Align your **thoughts** with the way you feel, or understand the emotions that lead to or lie underneath your thoughts

Stop experiencing emotions and feelings that are related to your **past**

Work with your emotions and feelings in ways that empower you

In your struggle, you may find that you:

Block your emotions and feelings, and you cannot move them

Bury your emotions and feelings because they are causing too much pain

Suppress your emotions so you do not acknowledge them or feel them

Repress your emotions and feelings, and so do not work with them

To **work with** your emotions means to

- acknowledge them
- accept them
- affirm them

To **work against** your emotions means to

- resist them
- reject them
- suppress them
- repress them
- bury them
- hide them
- dismiss them

- push them
- fight them
- neglect them
- guard them
- defend them

Your emotions and feelings are **messages**, a signal to you or a way of communicating to you. What do you think your emotions and feelings are communicating to you?

The tools for working with your emotional self

ACKNOWLEDGE
It is important to accept or admit the existence of your emotions. Acknowledge the truth.

When something is stirring inside of you, what is happening in mind and body?
Ask yourself:
How do I feel?

Allow space and time for the truth of your emotion to appear.

Use this space to:
Observe your emotions
Introspect – examine your emotions
Recognize – identify what is happening to you in mind/body

Practice: Observe sensations

As you feel an emotion or feeling stirring inside of your mind and body, observe what the sensation is like.

Is it uncomfortable or unpleasant?

Practice: Observe physical symptoms

See how your emotions or feelings influence your body – observe what is happening to your body.

Ask yourself:
What is happening to my heart?
What is happening to my breath?
What is happening to my muscles?

NB: If the sensation or physical symptom is extremely uncomfortable, and if it is intensifying while you are observing, then pause and come back to this at a later stage.

HOLD SPACE
Keep space in your mind to allow your emotions to appear and flow through you without resistance or struggle.

Do not resist, reject, suppress, repress, bury, hide, dismiss, push away or fight emotions.

Do not judge your feelings; allow them to be whatever they need to be.

Imagine you were sharing a deep personal truth or pain with someone and they looked at you and judged you for your truth – how would that make you feel? So, be aware that each time you judge your own emotions and feelings, you are doing exactly that to yourself.

OBSERVE YOUR EMOTIONAL STATE

What condition does your emotion or feeling place your mind and body in? As you feel an emotion or feeling, ask yourself:

What state am I in?

If you struggle to find the answer, ask yourself:
Do I feel good?
Do I feel neutral?
Do I feel bad?

USE THE DICTIONARY OF FEELINGS

The Dictionary of Feelings helps you to be aware of your emotions and feelings. It will help you understand their purpose, their meaning and their symptoms so you can create space for yourself and learn to sit with and work with your emotions and feelings. The dictionary will also help you to identify and name your feelings and emotions.

The dictionary is split into three parts:
If you feel good, go to the Positive section (Page 63–99).
If you feel neutral, go to the Neutral section (Page 105–108).
If you feel bad, go to the Negative section (Page 111–181).

FIND THE MEANING AND PURPOSE

Use the Dictionary of Feelings to help you understand the meaning and purpose of your emotions. It is important to try to find the **meaning** of your emotions and the **purpose** behind them – why you feel the way you feel.

UNDERSTAND YOUR BODY

Use the Dictionary of Feelings to be aware of how your emotions affect your body, inside and outside.

The dictionary will help you understand what is happening inside of your body when your mind feels a good or a bad emotion, or when you feel negative, neutral or positive – for example, what happens to your brain, heart, lungs or internal systems, or what chemicals get released in the brain and body.

Be aware that not everyone experiences physical symptoms in the same way.

RECEIVE THE MESSAGE

The message your emotions and feelings is sending you can be found in the Dictionary of Feelings. Allow yourself to receive the message because your emotions are trying to communicate something to you.

What is the message?
The dictionary breaks down your emotions into:

  Name
  Meaning
  Purpose

  For example:
  Name: Fear
  Meaning: A powerful state of mind and being that tells your mind and body that there is a threat that can be harmful or dangerous.
  Purpose: To help you be aware you are not safe; to help you stay alert so you can protect yourself from

harm and danger; to help steer you away from harmful or dangerous situations.

When you feel fear, your mind is telling you that there is a threat of danger and sends a **message** to your body to protect itself. When you feel fear, you are being told to stay alert so you can defend yourself or steer yourself away from harm and danger.

Practice: Affirm message

See the message and say it back to yourself loud and clear.
I feel – fear.
I feel – I am in danger.
I feel – I am not safe.

By affirming the message, you are:

- letting your mind and body know you have received the message and that you accept the message
- confirming and validating how you feel
- stepping into awareness and taking the step to work with your emotions instead of against them

THE POWER OF A NAME, A MEANING AND A PURPOSE

The power of finding the name, meaning and purpose of how you feel will help you to meet your emotions and feelings, and allow you to take that step so you can:
sit with them
be with them
and receive the message.

As you search inside yourself for the feeling and then search outside for the words in the Dictionary of Feelings, you are taking the simple step of helping move your emotions and feelings from out of your mind and body and into life, and you are now working with your emotions and feelings.

Go deeper. Move below the surface.

Life is not linear. Life doesn't always make sense, and neither do your emotions and feelings. Your emotions and feelings are not linear; they work in layers, move in circles and cycles, and move your mind and drive your body in and out of emotional states.

Your emotions and feelings also are not always created purely in the present moment; old emotions and feelings can rise to the surface from a previous time. They are asking to be seen and worked with. This is when deeper work can help you to step below the surface to see what needs healing, and which emotions and feelings need to be worked with.

Practice: Ask questions

Why?

One way to help yourself go below the surface and do deeper work is, every time you feel an emotion or feeling, and you see the message it is sending you, ask yourself:

Why do I feel this way?
Is it old or new?

In order to recognize if the emotion or feeling is new or if it is resurfacing from the past, ask yourself:

Is this feeling old or new?

Only you can know the truth.

Have I felt this way before?

To understand whether this emotion or feeling is being repeated again and again, ask yourself:

Have I felt this way before?

If the answer is *Yes* – and especially if the emotion or feeling keeps repeating and resurfacing and rising in the present moment – this is a sign that you need to look inside yourself.

Be aware: If the emotion is negative and causing triggers, discomfort and pain, you are being called to help yourself to heal or release what is inside of you.

Practice: Look inside *first*

Divert your mental attention inwards to see what is happening inside of you.

If an emotion or feeling has been felt in the past and keeps repeating – no matter where your mind and body move in life – It is time to recognize that this is not happening outside you. Say:

This is inside of me.

By stating this, you will take your mental attention away from the outside and move your attention to your inside world, which is where the work needs to be done. Say:

I need to do the work.

The work means looking inside yourself for what needs attention, healing, releasing, changing – instead of searching outside or expecting the outside to change. If you are looking outwards for a change and somehow it does change your way for a while, this may help you in the short term but not in the long term, as the emotions and feelings are still inside of you, waiting to rise again. You will keep feeling the same way.

Practice: One step at a time

Working on the inside needs to be done slowly and carefully, allowing yourself just one step at a time, a little at a time, not rushing.

Allow your emotions and feelings to rise naturally as you experience life. Do not deny them, suppress them, or try to manipulate them. If you wait for them, expect them or demand them, you will block yourself from meeting the truth of how you feel. Affirming one step at a time will help you to relax and open your mind; and when your emotions naturally appear, be ready to meet them.

Always create time and space for yourself emotionally and use the Dictionary of Feelings to help you to see them, know them and understand them.

Practice: Recognize the layers

Emotions and feelings layer themselves one over the other and over the root, which is the truth underneath all the layers that are trying to help you to make it through.

What lies underneath?

Your emotions and feelings work in layers, which means it is important to be aware of the layers.

Each time you experience an emotion or feeling, ask yourself:

What lies underneath?

For example:
Underneath anger is hate
Underneath hate is hurt
Underneath hurt is the root cause, fear.
So, at the root of your anger is fear. Are you threatened in some way, or scared?

For example:
Underneath stress and pressure is frustration.
Underneath frustration is fear.
So, you are stressed because you are scared or because you are protecting yourself from threat or danger. Are you scared something will happen underneath the stress?

For example:
Underneath the mask of confidence is anxiety.
Underneath anxiety is fear.
So, you are scared. What are you scared of? Do you really feel confident, or is it just an act?

This means you are not in alignment with your whole self, only a part of yourself; you will not feel whole.

Practice: Work through the layers

Work with the layers, one step at a time. If you are experiencing many emotions at once, create space for yourself, and allow room for them to appear one at a time.

One layer at a time.

Practice: Reveal the root

There are four emotions that lie at the root of all the emotional layers.

At the root of positive emotions are joy and unconditional love.

At the root of negative emotions are fear and sadness.

The roots are the first emotions that lead you into or out of an emotional state, be it positive or negative. If you can get to a space where you are able to reveal the negative root emotion – the fear or the sadness – then this is the place where you will find your truth, and this is when you will have the power to change, transform, heal and move on.

If you can acknowledge, work with and release the fear and sadness inside, you will find it easier to feel joy again, and the unconditional love of life that comes with being alive and experiencing life.

If you can reveal joy and unconditional love, you will be connected to life and find it easier to be in a positive emotional state.

USE THE DICTIONARY OF FEELINGS
The Dictionary of Feelings lists 50 positive emotions and feelings.

- Read them.

- See them.
- Know them.
- Understand them.
- Be aware of them.

And then when you experience a positive emotion, you can recognize it and meet it.

The Dictionary of Feelings lists three **neutral** emotions that place your mind and body into a neutral state.
- Read them.
- See them.
- Know them.
- Understand them.
- Be aware of them.

And then, when you experience a neutral emotion, you can recognize it and meet it.

The Dictionary of Feelings lists 87 **negative** emotions and feelings that can push your mind and body into a negative state.
- Read them.
- See them.
- Know them.
- Understand them.
- Be aware of them.

And then when you experience a negative emotion, you can recognize it and meet it.

Emotional reactions

WORKING WITH EMOTIONAL REACTIONS

To be able to work with the way you internally react to energy, emotions, feelings, senses, sensations and vibrations that are moving inside of you, and see how you react, you need to become aware of your reactions through **observation** and **introspection**.

Observing your reaction means that you look closely at the way you react to the emotions, thoughts and feelings inside of you, or to the situations you are placed in or experience.

Introspection means your analysis of what you become when you react to them.

- What is your reaction?
- Does it feel mild?
- Does it feel balanced?
- Does it feel strong?

Be aware – if the reaction feels intense and strong, it is likely to be connected to a past experience.

At the end of each entry in the Dictionary of Feelings, the likely reaction(s) to that emotion is/are listed. This is to help you to understand what reactions to expect when your mind and body are in a certain emotional state.

For example, when your mind and body feel positive, it is natural to open up, accept, embrace and trust.

Positive emotions and feelings push your mind and body into a positive state and help you to connect with life and love. This is why you react this way.

When your mind and body feel negative, it is natural to close up, defend, reject, resist and mistrust.

Negative emotions and feelings push your mind and body into a negative state, trigger alarm bells and cause discomfort and pain. This is why you will react this way.

CHANGE HOW YOU REACT

Every individual is unique, no reaction can be guaranteed. It is therefore important you observe, introspect and recognize when your mind and body fall into a positive, neutral or negative state and observe your personal reactions to how you feel in your mind and body.

How do you react?

What is happening to you?

PAUSE. Instead of unconsciously reacting and acting as usual in an automatic or unconscious way, before you react and act, try to **pause** and create a space between the emotion and the reaction.

It is in this space you create between the emotion and the reaction that you will really see what is happening to you on both the inside and the outside. This is where your power lies.

Practice: Journal your reactions

If you need help to understand your reactions, get a notebook and start an emotional reaction journal. Writing down in words how you react on the inside or outside when your mind and body experience an emotion, feeling or sensation will help with change and healing.

Every time you experience an emotion or feeling – positive or negative – observe how you react.

Your reaction may be internal and/or external.

An internal reaction is when you have a mental reaction towards the emotions, feelings or any form of sensation you have come into contact with. You feel it, you react to it.

An external reaction is when your body feels the internal reaction or feels the emotion or feeling and is driven to move, act, reject or express the emotion of feeling.

It is important to see how you react, as the emotional reactions in life are where the largest change or healing or transformation takes place.

Ask yourself:
Is this reaction helping me?
Do I want to keep reacting this way?

This is the moment when you can create:
A **chance** for something to happen.
A **choice** about which way you can be or go.
A **change** to a different way.

Struggling with your emotions – alarms, triggers, red flags

It is important to pay attention to and work with the painful sensations and experiences – alarms, triggers, red flags – inside your body, as they signal possible threat, harm and danger. They are also a sign that something inside you from a past time – an old emotional wound – needs working through and healing, especially if your internal reactions are negative, strong and painful, are repeated to you often, and you are at a time in your life when you are not in danger, yet you still feel unsafe. This means you have not healed from the past experience, and as time goes by the trigger repeats and gets louder. You need to know that negative internal alerts, alarms, triggers and red flags, although uncomfortable and painful, are here to help you.

> Be aware: triggers reveal hurt and pain and what needs to heal.

The louder and stronger they are, the more they need to be worked with, as they are a clear sign that this is where the healing inside you needs to be done. Something inside of you is guiding you to heal.

WHAT HAPPENS WHEN YOU ARE "TRIGGERED"?

The trigger will cause your mind and body to feel like you are back in the same time and place where the past hurt occurred – it takes your mind and body out of the present moment. You will relive the same mental, emotional and physical symptoms, only with time these symptoms can become louder and more painful. You will hurt inside, and with this pain you will not be able to see or hear yourself or differentiate if this experience is from the past or is still in the present.

If you are unaware this is happening, you may find yourself fighting against the trigger and the emotions that have resurfaced inside of you. This can cause you to struggle and mentally and emotionally spiral backwards. This is why you must start to understand and recognize your own personal triggers – they are your internal guides to healing and evolving.

WHY DOES THIS HAPPEN?

Your trigger is asking to be seen and heard. There is something inside of you that is asking to be seen and heard and healed and released. It is signalling that it is time for you to do some inner work.

WORKING WITH YOUR TRIGGERS

Rather than ignoring the triggers and pain inside of you, and working against them, see them as friends with healing messages.

Your triggers are your internal guides to healing. If you see them as a friend and not an enemy when they appear inside of you, they will guide you and lead you to the exact place that needs healing.

If your trigger is based on a past experience, it will guide you to the hurt that keeps reappearing inside of you, which is causing you to struggle and react in negative ways and thus is holding you back. The past hurt is keeping you stuck in a cycle that you need to break free of. Your trigger guides you to the place you need to heal, so you can break free of this circle. Your triggers are your most prominent healers in life.

Be aware, if you do not become friends with your triggers or know how to work successfully with them, you will continue to experience past hurts, which can cause you to move deeper into a negative state, and this is when you can lose yourself in life. Your triggers will start to feel like enemies, as you think they are hurting you – they are not hurting you; they want to work with you and guide you.

Be aware, if you are experiencing very strong negative triggers and internal negative reactions, then this is a sign that you need to work through the layers of emotions to get to the root – please seek professional help.

Practice: Journal your triggers

It is essential that you keep a record of the times you are triggered and what follows.

If you feel yourself mentally or emotionally spiralling backward, or you feel that sudden pull inside of you before you start to spiral, pause and take a moment to look inwards – what is happening to you?

Ask yourself:

Where am I ?
Who am I with?
What position am I in?
How do I feel?
What are the emotions involved?
What is the negative narrative attached?

Pay attention.

Use the Dictionary of Feelings to help you understand the emotions that keep being triggered and need healing.

NEGATIVE EMOTIONAL SPIRALS

A negative emotional spiral is when you can feel your mind slipping backward into a negative space or place. Very quickly it can feel out of your control.

The spiral is a chain of emotions connected from one event to another based on your past experiences. This chain of negative emotions is attached and connected to past life experiences events, situations, circumstances and outcomes.

As your mind moves backward, all the old emotions, feelings, thoughts, beliefs, opinions, conclusions and sensations from your past will rise inside of you. If there are unhealed wounds that lie inside of you, there will be further triggers that will rise too.

Your mind has moved out of the present, and back into another space and place towards another time connected to your previous experiences and past events.

Practice: Stop negative emotional spirals

You must become aware of this spiral, as it can lead you down a very dark path. To stop you from spiralling, you need to say in a loud and clear voice:

STOP.

This should bring your mind and body back into the present.

Or you can stamp your feet ten times, or tap your face, or wash your face in cold water and bring your mind and body back into the present moment.

Use your physical body to bring you back to the present.

Loudly affirm: *I am in the present*.

You can also use your senses to bring you back to the present – try to name what you can see, hear, smell, taste and touch. Be firm on yourself, as if you are your very own stern parent. You know where this spiral will lead you, and you need to take care of your mental self and practise being mindful every day.

It is advisable, when the time is right, to revisit Chapter 2 to help you understand yourself inside and out and to be aware of why your mind spirals backward. Remember to keep a journal of the emotions leading you back to a particular time and place, and seek professional help so you can work with and release the feelings.

Negative cycles, circles, patterns

A negative cycle is a series of negative emotions that are regularly repeated in the same order.

A negative circle is a series of emotions that move in a loop and bring you back to the same starting point.

A negative pattern is a repeated way of being – the same reactions repeated in the same way so it makes a pattern.

These make you feel as if you are stuck in the same space, repeating the same experiences, and bring hurt, discomfort and pain. They can cause you to move further and further into a deep negative state, and this is when you can lose yourself in life.

The only way to break out of a negative pattern, cycle or circle is to change what is happening inside of you first – change the reaction or the way you act, or work with the emotions or feelings that keep repeating inside.

The change is on the inside.

Practice: Seven steps to break the cycle, circle or pattern

1. Recognize your cycle, circle or pattern.

Be aware that you are stuck in a cycle, circle or pattern and identify it.

Do you relate to the following?

- I feel stuck
- Outside events keep repeating
- Nothing seems to change

Ask yourself:

- Do the same thoughts keep repeating?

If the answer is _Yes, and it feels bad_, you are in a negative cycle, circle or pattern.

CHECK-IN: NEGATIVE CYCLES

Check inwards to identify which negative emotions and feelings keep repeating.
- Which emotions keep repeating?
- Make a list
- Use the dictionary

---

2. The negative narrative

Look inwards to see the story that keeps repeating inside of your mind and fuelling the fire.

What words or stories keep repeating?

3. Observe your reactions:

Note the way you react to negative energy, emotions, feelings, thoughts, sensations and vibrations.

Ask yourself: What do I keep doing the same?

EXERCISE: KEEP A JOURNAL

In this journal, write down all the negative emotions, feelings and thoughts that keep repeating. Noting the words attached to the feelings, it is important for you to be able to analyse your cycle, circle or pattern so you can break that link inside of you that keeps the connection to the cycle, circle or pattern.

Break the chain.

---

4. Create a space in between

Instead of reacting and acting as you do in your usual way, or in an automatic or unconscious way, pause and create a space in between the emotion and the reaction.

Pause before you react.

You have now created space for:

A chance for something different to happen.

A choice about which way you want to be or go.

A change in what happens next.

5. Find your core

Your core is the central part or who you are and the central part of your existence. It is the part of you that will stay constant; it is the truth of who you are.

To find your core and align with it, ask yourself:

Which reaction is no longer serving me?
Which reaction is not in alignment with me?
Which reaction is fighting for me in life, but no longer needs to?

Revisit Chapter 1, The Path of Empowerment, The Path of Destruction.

6. Create a change

To break the emotional cycle, circle or pattern, you have to break, erase or step out of it by making a move in a new direction – by changing the way you react internally.

Affirm: _I will create a change_.

Emotional pain and blockages

Emotional Pain: A negative state of mind and being that causes pain

Emotional Wounds: A negative experience that causes a deep pain

Emotional pain (negative state of mind) and emotional wounds (negative past experiences) are the hardest things to work through in life, as you cannot physically see your emotions, yet they keep hurting you again and again. Emotional pain, if not healed, can keep you stuck and blocked. You will find it hard to **move through** the pain because of the trigger inside you that brings you back to the same place.

Practice: Five steps to deal with your emotional pain

1. Acknowledge the truth
Ask yourself:
What is happening to me:
Mentally
Emotionally
Physically
Spiritually?

2. Sit with the truth
Use the Dictionary of Feelings to find which emotions are causing you pain.
Find them and sit with them. Acknowledge each one.
Do not stay there for too long, just greet and meet the truth.
There is a message in your pain and it needs to be seen.

3. Work through layers
How many emotions and feelings are attached to this pain?
Use the Dictionary of Feelings to work through the layers, along with the help of a friend or professional.

4. Reveal the root

What is the root emotion that lies beneath this pain?
Did it start with fear or with sadness?

MOVE YOUR FEELINGS AND EMOTIONS FROM THE INSIDE OUT.

5. Express your emotion

Ways in which you can express the energy, emotion or feeling stirring inside of you include:

Words: Use spoken or written communication to reveal the truth of how you feel

Dancing: Use music and movement to see, feel and release your emotions

Movement: Mentally, emotionally, physically and spiritually move to a new place

Tears: Cry to release pent-up internal emotions

Exercise: Acknowledge the emotion and work through it physically

Energy work: Professional therapists can help you to release the energy inside

Express.

Be aware, if you do not express your emotional energy, feelings and thoughts, they can weigh your mind and body down. You can get lost inside them, which will keep you struggling in negative patterns, cycles and circles, and will also block your spirit, which is the part of you that is connected to life. Find a way to release the truth of how you feel inside to a place outside of you.

Practice: Communicate the unseen, the unspoken, the unexpressed, the unrevealed

Say:

I feel ... (name the emotion)

I feel uncomfortable (explain why)

I feel stuck in a ... (name the pattern, circle, cycle)

I feel ... (name the trigger), and I do not know why.

I feel love for ... (be honest with this feeling)

I feel as if I am going through ... (name the thing)

I feel I need help to help me work with my inner world.

EMOTIONAL CHECK-IN

Check in with yourself emotionally.

If you are an adult, you have come a long way in your life. You have felt your way through life from the day you were born to where you are now. You have emotionally and energetically absorbed life inside of you and outside of you. You have had to find a way to figure life out, and learned how to work with your own emotions and feelings, as well as try and understand other people's. You also may have picked up emotions and feelings that did not belong to you, and carried emotional pain that was not yours, yet you carried on. You were not given a guidebook in life regarding how to work with your emotions, yet here you are. You came through.

EXERCISE: EMOTIONAL CHECK-IN

Close your eyes
Ask yourself:
- How are you?
- How are you feeling?

Make these statements:
- I see you.
- I understand you.

11

HOW TO SUCCESSFULLY WORK WITH YOUR PHYSICAL SELF

Step 4: Learn how to work "with" and not "against" your physical self.

Physical self

Your body is miraculous and powerful. From birth, it connects you to the world, and helps you to move through life. Your body represents you on the outside. Without your body, you would not be here. It is the part of you that feels and explores, and identifies and creates who you are in being. Your physical body is significant, and your inner body, which has over 12 systems, is mind-blowing.

Within your physical body are the following systems:

Muscular

Skeletal

Nervous

Endocrine

Cardiovascular

Integumentary

Immune

Respiratory
Digestive
Urinary
Lymphatic
Reproductive

However, your body is not the only part of you. Your body is also connected to the other nine parts of you:

Mind
Spirit
Instincts
Senses
Emotions
Feelings
Reactions
Actions
Behaviour

If all the parts are not aligned, your body will be out of balance.

Your physical body creates and holds:
Energy
Emotions
Feelings
Instincts
Sensations
Memories
Thoughts

Your physical body on the outside is expressed as:
Shape
Size
Skin colour
Hair colour and texture
Eye colour and shape
Gender – male or female

Your physical senses use your:
eyes (sight)
ears (hearing)
nose (smell)
mouth (taste)
hands (touch)

Your senses:
identify (recognize and understand)
explore (travel and learn)
perceive (become aware and conscious using our senses)
percept (understand in your way)

What impacts the physical self?

Internal physical condition: Is it healthy or unhealthy?
External physical condition: Is it healthy or unhealthy?
Mind: How you think about your physical self (thoughts, beliefs, judgements)?
Mind: How you think about others' physical selves (thoughts, beliefs, judgements)?

Feel: How you feel about yourself physically (emotions and feelings)?

Feel: How others feel about you physically (emotions and feelings)?

Nutrition: Is the food you put in your body balanced, healthy, nutritious?

Self-care: How do you maintain and cleanse your body? Do you engage in self-care?

Movement: Do you move your body? Is it fit and flexible?

The physical struggle

If you struggle physically, then you may struggle to connect with, or work with, or just be yourself physically. You may have negative emotions and thoughts about your physical self, and/or feel bad internally or externally. Your physical body may not be in a healthy or strong state and needs to heal.

You may react to these struggles in ways that are not the truth of who you are. You may refuse to accept parts of your physical self, and reject, neglect or even hurt parts of your physical self. You may act in ways that are not your true self and are far away from your core.

You may struggle with your appearance, shape or size, your colour or your gender.

In response, you may have unhealthy reactions, actions and behaviours, which create an unhealthy body and mind. You may engage in abnormal, addictive, aggressive or distracted behaviour or self-sabotaging habits or patterns. You may also have destructive habits, patterns or behaviours.

The tools for working with your physical self

Your first tool will be a pen and notebook. In your notebook write the title *My Physical Self*, then make notes as instructed below.

ACKNOWLEDGE
It is important to accept yourself physically. Ask yourself:

Who am I?

Practice: See your true self

Look at your physical self in a mirror.
   Find a place where you can see your whole physical – preferably in a full-length mirror.
   Wear either a thin layer of clothes so that you can see your body shape, or not clothes at all.
   You must not hide behind your clothes.

   When you are ready, you need to look at your true physical self clearly.
   Set an alarm clock, and look at yourself in the mirror for one full minute.
   In this one minute, observe all that you are physically.
   What do you see?

- Shape?
- Size?
- Colour?
- Features?

- Do you have scars?
- Do you have flaws?

Move closer to the mirror.
Do you feel comfortable or uncomfortable?
Move even closer.
Look into your eyes.
What do you see?
When the one minute is over, move back to a place where you are comfortable.
Put on clothes that you feel comfortable in.

Get your pen and paper and answer the following questions:
Am I comfortable or uncomfortable looking at myself?
Do I like what I see?

If the answer is <u>*Yes*</u>, write down what it is you like instantly, without delay.
Write down the good thoughts that entered your mind when you saw yourself.

If the answer is <u>No</u>, then ask: <u>*Why not?*</u>

Write down what you see and feel immediately, without delay or thinking.
Write down the bad thoughts that entered your mind when you saw yourself.

Be honest. Do not hide behind lies. This is an exercise to see your true self, to get to the root of how you really feel about your physical self. Be truthful to yourself.

CHECK IN: WHERE AM I IN LIFE?

Think about where are you physically in your life. Get a pen and paper and jot down your answers to the following questions.

How do I feel physically, both inside and outside?
Where am I?
What stage of life am I in?

Stages and Ages:

New-born:	0–1 years
Infancy:	1–2 years
Toddler:	2–4 years
Childhood:	4–11 years
Adolescence:	12–19 years
Adulthood:	20–40 years
Middle age:	40–60 years
Senior:	60–80 years
Advanced senior:	80+ years

What place am I in?
What position am I in?
Do I like my position in life?

If the answer is *No*, why not? What is happening to you in life that you don't like?

Also, in what position do you want to be in life?

When you have answered these questions, put a date and time against your answers. Put the paper away and do not look at it for a while.

Practice: Accept

You need to accept who you are and where you are for now, without resistance or struggle.

Acceptance allows your body to surrender in the present time without resisting, fighting, struggling and pushing. Acceptance will create space inside of you. It will free up the energy used to resist, fight, struggle, push, and allow yourself to be as you are.

Give your mind permission to stop overworking and struggling. This is when you can use the space you have just created for yourself as a way to help you to see clearly where you are in life, what you are going through, and what is happening inside and outside of you.

Use the space you have just freed up to create change.

Before you change, accept yourself.

Practice: Affirmations

Take time to create space for yourself and mentally accept who you are.

Find time to sit with yourself
In a safe and comfortable place
Breathe
In
Breathe
Out

When you are ready
Affirm: *I accept who I am.*

EXERCISE: SIMPLY BE

This is a 14-day, five-step exercise where you will simply be in your body, and move with the flow of life.

Now that you have accepted your physical self, and affirmed this acceptance in your mind, over the next 14 days, you will take five steps that will help you to simply be in your body. It is important you take these five steps if you want to make any change in the future. Mark "simply be" on your calendar for the next 14 days.

To "simply be" is that moment when you are fully present in your body, using all five of your senses to fully appreciate where you are in life, to fully appreciate your experience of life and being alive in your body, and to fully accept yourself for who you are.

1. Simple pleasures

Being mindful and enjoying the simple pleasures that life brings, living life in the moment, helps you to connect to joy and can create positive feelings that come with simply being – and enjoying the pleasures of life.

Each day, try something like one of the following:
-preparing a special drink
-cooking your favourite food
-being with family
-being with a friend
-doing a hobby
-playing or listening to music
-painting or drawing

If you do not know what your simple pleasure is, ask yourself: What is my simple pleasure?

Then write down five pleasures that come to mind, and over the next 14 days make time for yourself to simply enjoy them. Fully embrace where you are, who you are with, what is happening, and trust deep down inside of you that everything will be okay.

2. Use all your senses

Use all five senses to fully connect to life in the moment:

Eyes to clearly see the world around you.
Ears to simply listen to the sounds around you.
Nose to smell the fragrances around you.
Mouth to taste the flavours or your meals.
Touch to feel the textures around you.

In the next 14 days, you will use all of your senses to see, hear, smell, taste, touch or feel and connect to your present moment. For example, if you go outdoors, allow your senses to see the green, to listen to the sounds of birds, to smell the flowers, to feel breeze on your skin.

If you connect with a loved one during the 14 days, try to see them deeply, without judging how you think they should be.

Keep your mind still for 14 days and take the opportunity to see, hear, smell, taste and touch the experience of your life and body and those of your loved ones.

Take the chance to smile at another person – truly smile – and see how that feels to you on the outside. From your eyes, your smile rises.

3. Ground the soles of your feet

This is a therapeutic technique that allows you to realign your mind, body and spirit to the earth.

Over the next 14 days, make sure you walk barefoot on cold ground or earth. Step outside of your mind and into your body, allowing yourself to be balanced and aligned.

4. Connect to nature

Nature can help you ground yourself and allow you to step into your entire being. The earth will also help you to release the energy or emotions that are stirring inside of you, or help you erase the narratives you are creating.

Nature means the earth, the sky, the sun, the wind, the rain, the trees, the rivers and lakes, the sea, the rocks, the plants, the breeze, the animals, and all that is natural in life.

As you connect to nature, let go and surrender your physical self.

Take deep breaths of outside air, do not resist.

Allow the sun's rays to meet your skin, even for a short while.

Allow your skin to feel the breeze.

Allow your eyes to see the beauty that nature provides.

Allow your ears to hear the birds and sounds of life.

Allow your hands to feel the bark of a tree.

Feel all that energy that is stirring inside of you leave your body and move into the earth.

Connecting to nature is important, especially if your body is imbalanced and your mind and body are experiencing turbulent emotions. Nature helps to balance your body, which can help your body move back into a homeostasis state. A homeostasis state is when your body is in a state of balance, and all the internal organs and systems are moving as they should, in harmony.

5. Simple Observation

Observe yourself with a silent mind; do not use your mind to control your life with a narrative that it should be like this or like that, or to judge how it should be – allow it to unfold without any controls.

Over the next 14 days, start to observe your physical self – just be yourself and observe.

And ask yourself:

- How do I act?
- How do I react?
- How do I behave?
- Is my behaviour natural?
- Is my behaviour learned?
- Is my behaviour masked?

You can also ask yourself:

What is my persona (the way my character is perceived by others) like?

What is my character (the nature of me, the way I am formed) like?

What is my personality (the combination of characteristics that form my unique character) like?

Make written notes of what you do not like about what you have observed, and add this to the other notes in your "Physical" folder.

EXERCISE: REVIEW

Now is the time to review your truth. Make sure you have some time when you won't be disturbed and are in a safe space. When you are ready, open up your notes on *My Physical Self*.

How many **positives** were there? *I feel good about my physical self*.
How many **neutrals** were there? *I feel okay about my physical self*.
How many **negatives** were there? *I feel bad about my physical self*.

Look at the things you felt negative about and ask yourself: *Can I change it?*

Are you in a position to change it?
If the answer is *No*, then ask yourself:
Can I change how I feel about it?
Can I work with my negative feelings so I do not keep feeling bad?
Use the Dictionary of Feelings.

If the answer was *Yes, I can change it*, the next question to ask yourself is:
Do I WANT to change it?

In order to make a change, not only do you have to accept yourself as you are now and what is happening to you, it is vitally important that you **want** to change.

NB: If you did not make notes as you worked through this chapter, go back to the beginning and start the process again. It is important you do this if you want to make any changes or transformations to your physical self, or make any changes to how you feel about yourself.

Practice: Physical change and transformation

Change means to make something new or different.
   Transformation means to change in appearance, character, personality or behaviour.

   Change and transformation have to happen slowly and carefully, un-rushed, one step at a time.
   Change starts with one small act, which will contribute toward creating change.
   The act that you choose to make has to be a new act, which helps you take that step towards change.

1. **Be clear about what you want to change**
   Sit down with a pen and paper, write down the title *My Physical Change.*
   In a calm quiet space, when you are ready, ask yourself:

   What do I want to change?
   I want to change...
   I want to change this because...

2. Use the power of your mind

Your mind is a powerful force, use its vision and imagination.

**See it before you achieve it.
Envision the change.**

If you are finding it hard to envision the change, collect images to inspire you. Put these images in one place, and every time you feel like moving back into a familiar place, or you can no longer see the vision, look at the images and ask:

How do the images make me feel?

3. Imagine your future self

Imagination is when you use the power of your mind to envisage what you want; it can be so powerful that you can see it and feel it, and believe it is there in your mind. The power of imagination is that it can take you anywhere in your mind, and your vision can be anything you want it to be.

Imagine yourself in the future when the transformation is complete.

Set aside 15 minutes in the morning and 15 minutes in the evening and, for the next 14 days, imagine your transformation.

Close your eyes
Breathe naturally
Place your hand on your heart
What do I want to change?
Can I see it in my mind?
Do I believe it can happen?

Allow your mind to create a vision
How do I feel?
How do I want to feel?
How do I look?
How am I moving?

4. **Take a physical step**

In your notebook, title this *A New Change*.

In this step, make sure you physically:

Create a goal – What is your goal? What needs to change?

Prepare – What do you need to achieve this goal?

Plan – What actions need to be taken to get to the end goal?

Create mini goals – Have something small and easy to reach for, to help you get to the final result.

5. **One new action**

To keep moving towards the change, take one new action at a time.

For example, if your goal was:

I want to change my body shape.
I want to change my body image.
I want to change my bad habits.

Ask yourself:

> What new action can I take?

6. **Power of elimination**

If you do not need a new action, and you simply need to change habits that are no longer serving you in life, you can try something even more powerful that can help you – the **power of elimination**.

Eliminate an old action: To keep moving toward the change, remove an old action.

Just for one day, stop doing an old action.

As the day comes to an end and you are ready to go to sleep at night, congratulate yourself and promise you will do the same for yourself the very next day.

Then repeat the elimination to keep moving toward the change. Continue to honour this new routine for the next week.

More tools for working with your physical self

MOVEMENT

Move your physical body into a positive state. Move your body to release the old energy of yesterday and create new, positive energy and emotions that help you feel good.

When you make a personal choice to take action to move your body into a new state, you are choosing to help your mind and body to move out of an old state and into a new state. This choice can help your mind and body release the natural feel-good chemicals inside of you:

Dopamine: a chemical in the brain that helps you with reward, motivation, memory and attention

Endorphins: hormones released in body to help relieve pain and stress

Serotonin: a chemical in the brain that helps lift mood, and with digestion and sleep

Moving your body can also help boost your body's internal systems, which work 24 hours a day to help keep you alive.

For example, through movement you will boost your circulatory system, which is responsible for pumping oxygen into your heart and lungs and circulating blood through the body; you will strengthen your immune system, which is responsible for defence and protection; and you will improve your respiratory system, which circulates oxygen to your lungs and helps you breath.

It is important you seek medical advice before starting any new exercise regime.

Ways to move your body to help improve physical fitness and wellbeing include:

Walking at a regular pace

Dancing formally or informally

Sport, be it for fun or competitively.

As you move your body, make sure you work on your **core** – the physical centre which is also central to your existence, and your **muscles** – your physical power and strength.

NOURISH YOUR BODY WITH JOY

Ensure that you eat food that nourishes your body, but also that whatever you eat, you eat it with joy. Joy is a positive state of mind that connects you to the joy of life; when you make a choice to eat with joy, you are honouring your body and honouring the experience of life.

To nourish your body means to eat in a way that honours your body; it means to:
eat well, in a way that satisfies you
eat healthily, in a way that promotes a healthy body and wellbeing
eat nutrients, which are essential for growth
eat natural antibiotics to help protect your body

Using your physical senses to see, smell, touch and taste food is one of life's greatest pleasures. Food can nourish the body, stimulate your senses, unite your mind and body, and also help you connect with loved ones.

Affirm: _I choose to eat with joy_.

Practice: One bottle of water

Hydrate and cleanse your body, and eliminate toxins.
Find a water bottle, and make sure you drink a minimum of one full water bottle a day. As time goes on you can build this up to two, three, four, five or six bottles a day.

SELF-CARE
It is important to take care of yourself and your needs to make sure you are physically well as well as mentally and emotionally well. To be at your best, you must not neglect your own needs, which include:

Sleep – to make sure your body has enough sleep to recover and stay healthy and energized

Breaks – to take time away and have a break for yourself, so you can recuperate and re-energize

Personal boundaries – to create space for yourself so your energy is not taken by another

Personal hygiene – to keep your hands, head and body fresh and clean

Health check – to seek professional medical help to make sure you are well

Take time to sit with yourself and ask:
How can I take care of myself to make sure I am at my best?

Create a self-care plan, to ensure self-care is a priority in your everyday schedule.

PRACTICE UNCONDITIONAL LOVE

It is important to love your body unconditionally, without any judgement, without the influence of:

beliefs – a mental acceptance that the body should be this or that

opinions – your body as you see it based on your position and viewpoint

criticism – the expression of faults, flaws and mistakes

judgements – the conclusion that this is how it should be

expectations – a strong belief that beauty is a certain way

Unconditional love is a love so pure that it does not expect anything in return. It is to love your body for what it is – a part of you, a creation of you, which is with you on your journey of life. Unconditional love is to not allow the outside world to influence you or impact you or tell you how your body should be.

Say: *I love my body unconditionally.*

Life is precious and sacred and so is your body. It is up to you to choose to take care of it, love it and respect it.

CHECK-IN: YOUR PHYSICAL SELF

Use the power of your mind to check in on your physical self.

Before you go to sleep at night

Take 10 minutes of your time

Close your eyes

Breathe in deeply

Inhale

Exhale

When you are ready

Mentally scan your body

Connect to each physical part

Slowly move your mind through your body

Start with the tips of your toes

Slowly move your way up to the top of your head

Scan for areas of tension, pressure, pain or discomfort

How does your body feel to your mind?

Which parts are stimulated?

Which parts are blocked or shut down?

Are there emotions or tension stored inside you?

As you mentally move your mind to check in on your body, send your body some love:

Breathe into the areas that are tense, tight or feel painful, and then move on

When you get to your heart, send your heart love and healing and move up

When you get to the top of your body, take a few deep breaths, and slowly open your eyes

If something doesn't feel right in your body, always make sure you seek medical help or see an energy expert who can help you release stored energy in your body that may be trapped inside you.

CHECK-IN: PHYSICAL AND EMOTIONAL REACTIONS

It is important to be aware of how your body reacts to energy, emotions, feelings, thoughts, and triggers old emotional wounds that stir inside of you.

It is important you are aware of your internal reactions, as it is your internal reactions that drive your physical reactions, which lead to actions and behaviour. It is your internal reactions that you are left alone with at night in the dark. If your internal reactions are not worked with in a successful way or are not taken care of, or get dismissed or ignored, then your inner world will become harder to navigate, and then the emotional discomfort and pain inside of you will get louder and louder.

CHECK-IN: EMOTIONAL REACTION

How does the emotional reaction inside of you feel? Does it feel:

- light
- medium or
- strong?

The stronger the reaction the bigger the need to step into your inner world to find out what is happening inside of you. A strong reaction is a clear sign that something needs to be worked with, or there is something that needs to be revisited or relooked at, or that you need to create space inside of you for inner healing. This can be a result of old emotional wounds from your past, which are impacting your present moment in time.

How does your emotional reaction express itself on the outside?

As you feel an emotion or feeling, observe or introspect your reaction on the outside of yourself. Is your reaction:

-an underreaction,

-a balanced reaction or

-an overreaction?

UNDERREACTION

With an **underreaction**, you will have little or no reaction, even though that does not match the situation or event, but something inside of you is driving you to react or act in that way. This can be a sign that you are not sure what to do in a situation or have found a way to avoid, deny or bury what is happening to you.

Be aware: Burying your internal reactions, emotions, feelings and thoughts can lead to strong triggers that will become louder and feel more painful in time. It is essential you learn to react in a healthy and balanced way.

BALANCED REACTION

A **balanced reaction** means you are aware of how you feel on the inside of your body, and have seen your emotions, feelings and thoughts stirring and respond to the moment in an appropriate manner.

A balanced reaction requires some understanding of your feeling(s). It also requires an understanding of the whole situation. A balanced reaction is more of a response than a reaction, as you have gone within and viewed the situation from a new, evolved perspective. Your response matches the situation and does not allow the wounds of your past to impact your present.

OVERREACTION

An **overreaction** is extreme and overpowering; it is not balanced, and you will not have any control over your emotions or feelings. This is a sign that you are not being treated as you would like in life, and you feel the need to fight back. When you overreact, you lose complete control of yourself and the situation. You become so focused on reacting to what you are feeling inside and from a state that is uncomfortable for you, that you temporarily forget your surroundings and may even do something regretful or harmful.

Before you react, ask yourself:

> Am I reacting with love or fear?

This should help to realign you to your core and your true self, and to your whole self.

CHECK IN: PHYSICAL BEHAVIOUR

It is important to check in on yourself to see if your behaviour is aligned with your truth, and is in line with who you want to be in this life. Underneath every reaction and action and behaviour lies the truth of how you feel. Before you behave in a certain way, ask yourself:

Is this who I am?
Is the way I behave in life aligning with the truth of who I am?
Is my behaviour getting lost in positive or negative states, emotions or feelings?
Is my behaviour getting lost in fear? Do I feel safe?

STATEMENTS
Finally, to always make sure you are working successfully with your physical self, try making a clear statement to yourself and body.

> I will honor my body.
> I will listen to my body.

The mind–body–spirit connection

The mind–body–spirit is a connection that links one to another. It is important to be aware of and understand the mind – body – spirit connection; otherwise you will only be working with the mind and/or the body, leaving no room for your spirit.

12

HOW TO SUCCESSFULLY WORK WITH YOUR SPIRITUAL SELF

Step 4: Learn how to work "with" and not "against" your spiritual self.

Spiritual self

Your spirit is the unseen, powerful part of you that brings you to life, connects you to life and helps you feel that sacred energy of life. It is extremely important that you are connected with and work with your spiritual self, and that you do not neglect, block or disconnect your spirit in life. Your spirit works in alignment with your mind and your body. It helps you to move through emotions and feelings. It helps you to relook at or release the emotions and feelings, reactions and actions, and habits and patterns that are stuck in the body, still hurting you and holding you back in life. Your spirit brings you closer to life when you lose your way, and is the part of you that connects you to other forms of life and to the rest of humanity.

Your spirit can be blocked by:

- stuck emotions or feelings
- suppressed emotions
- repressed emotions
- buried emotions
- blocked emotions
- stuck beliefs
- fixed beliefs
- fixed thoughts
- fixed opinions
- fixed judgements
- fixed conclusions
- fixed view
- destructive reactions
- destructive actions
- destructive habits
- destructive patterns
- ego

What is ego?

The ego is the part of you that is strongly attached to your emotions and feelings, thoughts, opinions, judgements, conclusions and beliefs, and is the part of you that holds on tight to a narrative and cannot let go. The ego is also the part of you that is strongly attached to your physical identity.

This means your ego is the part of you that fights for:

status – an accepted or official position that places you in a social group

title – the name you call yourself

role – the position which you place yourself in life

The ego protects you and keeps you strong in life. If you are unaware of your ego and your ego is overused without your awareness, it can get in the way of your connection to your spirit. Your ego can separate you from yourself, it can separate you from others, and most of all it will disconnect you from what is important in life. If your ego is used unconsciously, it can prevent you from evolving in life and seeing life in a new way or from a new perspective or through a new lens, as what you need to see in order to evolve cannot be seen if the ego gets in the way. Eventually, if you need to evolve and you choose to stay stuck in your ego or fixed in your ways, repeating the same mistakes again, your spirit will break through and find a way to make you change, and this is when you can break.

The spiritual struggle

The spiritual struggle means:

You struggle with what you are perceiving in life, and thus disconnect. You struggle to feel, so you block, disconnect, bury, push away or reject. You create a reality and close your mind to other ways of thinking. Your overactive thoughts block out your spirit and block the spirit of life. You react and act in ways that only work with your physical self, rather than with your spiritual self also. You behave in ways that misalign with the truth of who you are in life.

Means: You struggle to connect with life, or to connect or feel the spirit of life

Perceive: You struggle with what or you are perceiving in life, and disconnect

Feel: You struggle to feel, you block, disconnect, bury, push away or reject

Think: You create a reality and close your mind to other ways of thinking

Thoughts: Your overactive thoughts block out your spirit and block the spirit of life

Reaction: You react in ways that only work with your physical self

Actions: You act in ways that only work with physical self

Behaviour: You behave in ways that misalign with the truth of who you are in life

Your spirit works in mysterious ways.

Tools for working with your spiritual self

ACKNOWLEDGE
It is important to acknowledge your spiritual self to accept and acknowledge that there is more to you than the physical self.

Affirm: *I am more than physical.*

Acknowledging your spirit will help you to let go of the parts of you that are blocking you from your spirit, or blocking you from evolving. It will also allow your emotions and feelings to move through your mind and body. Be aware: stuck emotions and feelings can block your spirit.

Make room for your spirit

Your emotions:
To help separate yourself from your emotions and feelings so you can see them and work with them and still be connected to your spirit, affirm:

I am not my emotions.

Your thoughts:
Do not get trapped in your thoughts or allow your thoughts to block your connection with your spirit.

To help separate yourself from your thoughts, so you can leave room for your spirit, affirm:

I am not my thoughts.

Your opinions:
An opinion is a judgement based on your personal position and point of view. It is not all of you. It is a part of you that can block your connection to your spirit.

Allow yourself to have an opinion and then separate yourself from the opinion and create space for your spirit. Affirm:

Affirm:

I am not my opinions.

Your beliefs:
A belief is created in your mind to give you meaning and purpose in life. A belief gives your mind something to hold on to. Your mind will attach itself to the belief and then keep reacting, acting and behaving in response to the belief, and will not see beyond the belief you have created in your mind. If you

stay firmly strong and fixed to beliefs, you can lose connection to your spirit and to life as a whole. Affirm:

I am not my beliefs.

Your mind:

Overthinking can block your connection with your spirit and life. To allow yourself to move beyond your thinking mind, affirm:

I am not what I think I am.

DO NOT HOLD ON TOO TIGHT.

ALLOW LIFE TO FLOW AND UNFOLD

It is important to help yourself let go of all that is in your mind and surrender your mind and body to your spirit and life. Do not always control life with your mind; allow life to flow and unfold (move and trust that it will guide you) in new ways.

> Allow life to unfold.

Affirm: *I am ready to trust and let go.*

NB: Only affirm this if you feel safe to do so. If you do not feel safe, seek help so you do feel safe.

Finally, allow your mind to rest, and allow your spirit to move through your mind and body and around you in life. As you do this, pay attention to where you are guided or what comes to you naturally, without any need to control. For example, listen to the lyrics of a song that you unexpectedly chose to listen to, or pay attention to the next movie you are drawn to watch and receive messages from the words. Pause for a moment when you receive a call from someone, or pay close attention when you bump into an old friend – why have these things suddenly fallen on your path? Open your mind to what life places on your path – look out for signs, coincidences and synchronicities (a series of events that align on the outside and speak to you on the inside) that lie beyond the noise of the mind. These signs, coincidences and synchronicities help you to see that there is more to life beyond the mind and body.

Ways to connect to your spirit

Practice: Creativity

Over a 14-day period, to learn to let go and be in a flow and connect to your spirit, schedule time to be creative. Try to:

Write from your heart and spirit, not from your mind; allow your hand and body to move freely.

Draw or paint a picture and allow yourself to express yourself without thinking, caring or judgement; allow your hand and body to move freely.

Close your eyes
Breathe
Inhale
Exhale
Go deep within

Connect to your spirit
Say to your spirit within:
Allow me to be creative today.

It is important you do not allow your mind to get in the way if you want to be creative. Allow your mind to take a back seat and trust your spirit to lead with these activities; surrender your mind and body and go with the flow; allow it to happen how it happens and let something inside of you guide you to **be free**, to be how you want to be, to be creative.

Make sure you prepare: gather all the tools you need and do not limit your time.

Give yourself space and time so you can keep going until something inside of you tells you you're done.

Practice: Dancing

Learn to let go and connect to your spirit through dancing, moving your body naturally to music or to the rhythm of life.
Choose a time in your schedule when you can let go of your mind and body and simply dance. When you dance, let your body move with your spirit. Allow yourself to move your body naturally without restricting yourself; listen deeply to sounds and vibrations of the music. Choose music that helps you to surrender and let go.
Dancing freestyle can help you to let go of all that is in your mind, and allow you to just be.

Practice: Music

Learn to let go and connect to your spirit through music. Allow your mind to rest and surrender to the music. As the music moves and flows through the mind and body and moves and flows through life, it can help your mind and body become unstuck and move through your energy, emotions and feelings. Music can also help release mind control and resistance and the need to always be overthinking. Most importantly it can help you connect to your spirit. If you can allow your spirit to guide you, you can create personal playlists for your life journey, and create a music compilation that can help you raise your vibration and elevate your mood.

Allow yourself to be guided to the right music; something inside your body will draw you into the music that speaks to your spirit. Do not choose music just because it is what everyone else likes; allow yourself to instinctively, intuitively listen to what naturally draws you in with a feeling or a sensation, or a sign from a lyric that connects you to your spirit within. Music is the essence of spirit.

Most of all, find time to...

BE SILENT

Silence the mind and still the body so you can connect to your spirit, connect to life and connect to the deepest part of who you are, and move beyond the layers and conditioning.

If you have not been taught how to connect to your spiritual self, you may find yourself moving through life on autopilot and only working with your mind and body. You may get to a space and place in life where something inside of you is calling you to go inwards, to heal what is inside of you or to release what no longer serves you in life. But if you are unaware of this – if you cannot hear this call – then you can start to become stuck or feel trapped. If you are stuck your mind will struggle to find a way to move, so it will just move to a familiar place, to a place it knows – to a place that is conditioned or to a place it has been taught. Over your life, you will have been taught who to be, what to be, how to be. There will be so many teachings that would have been passed down to you by others, by mentors, teachers, friends, family, and others.

Pay deep attention.

Practice: Sit in silence

Learn to sit with your mind, body and spirit in silence. Start with a minimum of 10 minutes a day, and build up to 30 minutes a day within 30 days.

Create a sacred place
A place you feel safe
A place you can relax
Sit in silence with yourself

The goal of sitting in silence is so you can move your mind to see beyond all that you see in the physical world, which can cause your mind to be in a certain state or place, or can condition your mind to be a certain way.

Sitting in silence will allow you to move beyond all the noise in the outside world and beyond the words and actions and teachings that are being presented to you on the outside in the physical world. It is so you can move beyond layers and layers of conditioning that has been passed down by your carers, teachers, mentors and previous generations at another time and place.

Most importantly, it is so you can come back to the truth of who you are and align with your whole self. It is in this silence that the truth of life lies, and it is with the truth of life your spirit resides.

> See beyond.

You can choose to sit in silence:
at home
in nature
outdoors
with your community

Listen to that silent space.
Be comfortable in silence.

Ask yourself:
What does my spirit say?

Practice: Singing

Singing helps you to connect to the essence of your spirit and releases what is inside of you.

Try singing:
Hymns – a spiritual song or poem
Mantras – words or sounds repeated to help release what is inside of you
Pop music – find a harmonious tune or lyrics that connect to your truth

Singing is the voice of your spirit, and can help you to release what is inside of you; find a place to release your voice where you feel safe.

Whenever you feel like singing, just do it – sing out loud, and be proud of your voice and life.

Practice: I surrender

This practice may not be for you if you are new to spirituality, and have not been taught how to surrender your mind and body to a higher power; or if you do not believe in a higher power; or if you are uncomfortable moving your mind to something that is unknown or unseen that lies beyond the physical world.

However, if you would like to try this practice, this is your chance to surrender all that you are experiencing in your mind and body to a higher power or into a sacred space just by expressing six simple words, either from within or out loud to yourself.

Close your eyes.
Place your hand on your heart
Affirm: *I surrender to a higher power.*

The words you speak help you move your emotions and feelings, your pain, your hurt inside of you, into another space. It helps you to lay the burdens of life at the doors of a holy and sacred and more powerful space. It also helps you to go within and to speak from a place of vulnerability, beyond ego, beyond thinking you can do this on your own; it helps you to surrender your mind and body to something more powerful in life, something above you.

If you affirm these words each day for 14 days, something should shift within you.

Practice: Ask for help

If you are struggling or feel weighed down in life; or if you have experienced traumatic events and feel burdened in your mind and body; it is okay to ask for help. One way to do this, is to turn to a higher power, surrender your mind and body to your spiritual part, and ask to be shown the way – or at least find a place to lay your pain so that your mind and body don't have to carry all the weight.

Close your eyes
Place your hand on your heart
Ask: _Guide me, show me the way._

This will help you to find a love or faith within and release the negative energy or feelings that build up inside of you, in your mind and in your body.

Tools for working with the painful parts of your spiritual self

SPIRITUAL AWAKENING AND SPIRITUAL GROWTH

Spiritual awakenings or spiritual growth are painful processes. They are a breakdown and destruction of all that you think you are or trying to be, all that you have created for yourself that you are not, and all that you have built up inside and outside of yourself to believe that you are.

A spiritual struggle happens when your spirit starts to move through you in a very powerful way because you are in misalignment, and your spirit has a strong desire to move you into alignment with who you are.

A person is forced to let go of all the anger, hurt and pain they have been holding on to and surrender to the great mystery of life. Whatever you are going through, let go and remind yourself who you really are: your spirit will always mysteriously remind you of your truth.

Practice: Unconditional love

There is a love so powerful and pure, which resides inside of your mind and body. This love is limitless and boundless and goes beyond space and time. It is a love that moves beyond this physical world. This love is unconditional love. unconditional love does not expect anything in return. It helps you to surrender to something more powerful than the material world.

Unconditional love is often buried beneath all our other feelings, especially underneath fear. As life happens and your mind and body experience anger, hurt, pain and hate, your mind can layer into negative states; it is easy for you to get lost and not feel any type of love in life, let alone unconditional love. However, it is there inside of you.

As a human being you are born with unconditional love. If it feels safe for you, thank your mind and body for trying to defend and protect you behind fear, and ask your inner self if it is safe for you to feel unconditional love. If you can feel it, you will start to see and feel and experience life in a new way. Unconditional love binds, unites and connects you to life, and it especially helps you to feel connection to your spirit.

Allow yourself to work with your spirit and move through and see beyond your:

Beliefs
Behaviour
Emotions
Feelings
Judgements
Thoughts
Opinions
Reactions
Viewpoints

These have been created in the mind, and they cause additional pain and suffering as they can block unconditional love. When you are stuck with any of the above, you will struggle and suffer more than is necessary – or you can lose your way. If you can start to see and feel unconditional love, it can help heal the mind and body and connect you to your spirit.

Dig deep, beneath all the emotional layers of pain.

This powerful emotional state lies beneath the layers of hurt, hate, stress, worry and pain that you have experienced in life. Once you start to learn to work with your emotions and feelings and work with your negative states, and learn to release what no longer serves you, unconditional love will reveal itself to you.

Practice: Unlearning

Be prepared to let go of all that you have learned in life.

Life sometimes feels like a trick: you spend an entire lifetime learning, and just when you come to that space where you think you know everything, something moves inside of you, moving all that you have learned aside and making you question all that you think you know. What is happening to you? This is your spirit inside of you awakening. It is asking you to create room inside of you, so you can evolve and see a new way of being. Always remember:

```
Mind Learns
Spirit Unlearns
```

SPIRITUAL CHECK-IN

Check in on yourself to see if you are connected to your spirit. Ask:

Do I feel my spirit?
Do I connect to life?
Do I flow with life?
Do I respect life?

13

HOW TO SUCCESSFULLY WORK WITH YOUR WHOLE SELF

Step 4: Learn how to work "with" and not "against" your whole self.

Whole self

> You know who you are.
> Only you have the answer.

You are now coming to the end of the holistic guide.

> How do you feel?

The Blank Canvas

It is time to bring together your blank canvases, so you can see your whole self: mentally, emotionally, physically and spiritually.

SACRED TIME AND SPACE

Choose a time where you have the space and you are
in a sacred space to not be interrupted. Collect all the blank
canvases on which you wrote your truth as you read this book.

Read your words.

What do you see when you read the words?

Do they relate to who you are?

Now ask yourself:

Is this who I am, inside and out?

Are my words in alignment?

Is this who I want to be?

Take time to see what is happening to you mentally and
emotionally in your life.

Step outside of yourself for a moment, and take a step back
and look at your whole self.

Ask yourself:

Do I feel good?

or

Do I feel bad?

If you want to explore yourself further or face some truths.

Ask yourself:

What position am I in?

What events or circumstances am I experiencing?

What cycle of emotions am I experiencing?

Use the positive, neutral and negative blank canvases to see the truth about how you feel.

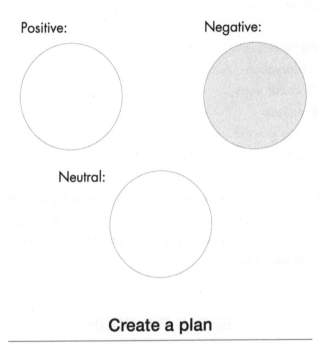

Positive:

Negative:

Neutral:

Create a plan

Once you have had time to see yourself inside and out, and have created and read over your blank canvases, create a plan for yourself:

> What do you want to change?

Is it your mental self, your emotional self, your physical self or your spiritual self? Or do you want to revamp, transform or change your whole self into a higher version of youself? Choose five new steps or practices from those recommended in Chapters 9, 10, 11 and 12. Which exercises, steps or practices reached out to you?

Which ones will help you move toward where you want to go in life?

Example:

1: Introspection
2: Observation
3: Practical steps
4: Exercises
5: Letting go and surrendering
6: Working with emotions or feelings

Implement five new steps, practices or exercises for 30 days.

After 30 days, add another two exercises or practices.

Start to practice a new way of being that feels in alignment with your whole self.

BREAK THROUGH

As you create this plan and see yourself inside and start the process of transforming and changing from old to new, make sure you especially focus on and take steps that will help you to break through all the parts that are holding you down and keeping you stuck; the parts that are struggling and reacting and disrupting; the parts that keep you in a negative cycle, circle or pattern; the parts that are no longer serving you or others or, in fact, the world.

Most importantly, break through the parts of you that keep reacting in old ways (on autopilot, and reacting in the same way again and again).

Make sure you change:

- old reactions
- old behaviours
- old habits

which no longer serve you in this life.

LIFE EXPERIENCE

Be aware: life will not always unfold in perfect ways. There will be days you will experience the unexpected, or days there may be no control, or days when you will make mistakes. If mistakes are made and you did not intentionally mean to make the mistake, or you lost your way, forgive yourself.

DO NOT KEEP REPEATING OLD MISTAKES.

LIFE LESSONS

What life lessons have I learned?

What lessons do I not want to repeat?

What can I do to make sure I do not repeat it?

DO NOT KEEP REPEATING OLD MISTAKES; this is what will hold you back in life. It is really important that you see your mistakes and you learn from your mistakes – grow with them and evolve through them so you can move forward and not hold yourself back. If you do not do this, life will have a mysterious way of bringing you back to the same space and place again until the lesson is seen and learned and worked... You may find yourself in a cycle and circle or feeling stuck because you are not seeing what you need to see in order for you to learn, evolve, and grow in life as a whole human being.

Take time to:

- pause
- reflect
- relook, re-examine
- relearn
- reset

... so you can always take time to step into alignment with your whole self.

After all, there will only ever be one version of who you are. You have come this far, and you only have the one life and one life experience. Be the best version of yourself there can be, and be the best version of yourself, inside and out.

CHECK-IN: WHOLE SELF

Check in with yourself to see if you are connected to your whole self. Ask:

What path am I on?

A path of empowerment?

or

A path of destruction?

Am I in alignment?
Is this who I am?

CHECK-IN: WHOLE SELF

Ask yourself:

How do I feel mentally?

How do I feel emotionally?

How do I feel physically?

How do I feel spiritually?

How do I feel as a whole?

Statements

Affirm:

I am more than.

I am whole.

I am a human being.

THANK YOU

Thank you for reading this guide. I hope it helped you to see parts of yourself that you have been struggling to see in yourself or work with.

I hope this guide has also inspired you to align with your whole self, and will help you to stop resisting and struggling,

I hope it will help you in the future as you make your way through life, and I hope it will help you to see your whole self, inside and out, even on days when you do not feel like yourself.

Life is a journey and an experience, and each and every person (including you) just wants to be seen, heard and understood. I hope you start to feel seen and understood, even if the person who sees you is you. That is who should see you.

Also be aware that as you move through stages, phases and places of your life, you may sometimes feel isolated or lonely. That is a normal part of life; you are not alone in feeling lonely on your journey. Each and every person on earth is travelling through this journey of life alone, in mind and body. Some days it is hard to describe what you are experiencing or going through... If you can, use the words in this guide to help you to express yourself, or release what is happening inside. It will help you to lighten up what you are experiencing, or help you to create space for yourself, so you can step into alignment with your whole self. It will help you to see your whole self, inside and out.

Always keep in mind that you are not just parts of yourself; you are more than you ever knew. There is power in all that you are. Do not disempower yourself – feel empowered.

Finally, I would like to thank the people in my life who saw me when I could not see myself:

My mother
My father
My siblings
My partner
My friends
My family
My colleagues
My neighbours
My community
My teachers in life (who ended up being children, especially D & D, my favourite mini teachers in life)
My publishers, especially R & K, who helped me bring this guide to life
Also, the stranger on the street who smiles at me
... and most of all I would like to thank myself: my mind, body and spirit, and my senses, my intuition, my emotions and feelings, for guiding me in this life. You helped me to step inside of my whole self, and when I have lost my way, your life gifts have always guided me back to my true self.

ABOUT CHERISH EDITIONS

Cherish Editions is a bespoke publishing service for authors of mental health, wellbeing and inspirational books.

As a division of Trigger Publishing, the UK's leading independent mental health and wellbeing publisher, we are experienced in creating and selling positive, responsible, important and inspirational books, which work to de-stigmatize the issues around mental health and improve the mental health and wellbeing of those who read our titles.

Founded by Adam Shaw, a mental health advocate, author and philanthropist, and leading psychologist Lauren Callaghan, Cherish Editions aims to publish books that provide advice, support and inspiration. We nurture our authors so that their stories can unfurl on the page, helping them to share their uplifting and moving stories.

Cherish Editions is unique in that a percentage of the profits from the sale of our books goes directly to leading mental health charity Shawmind, to deliver its vision to provide support for those experiencing mental ill health.

Find out more about Cherish Editions by visiting cherisheditions.com or by joining us on:
Twitter @cherisheditions
Facebook @cherisheditions
Instagram @cherisheditions

Cherish
EDITIONS

ABOUT SHAWMIND

A proportion of profits from the sale of all Trigger books go to their sister charity Shawmind, also founded by Adam Shaw and Lauren Callaghan. The charity aims to ensure that everyone has access to mental health resources whenever they need them.

You can find out more about the work Shawmind do by visiting shawmind.org or joining them on:

Twitter @Shaw_Mind
Facebook @ShawmindUK
Instagram @Shaw_Mind

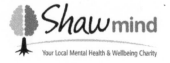

Your Local Mental Health & Wellbeing Charity